DIABETES

IN THE

FAMILY

Revised Edition

DIABETES

IN THE

FAMILY

Revised Edition

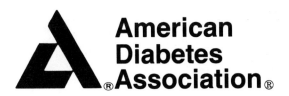
American
Diabetes
Association

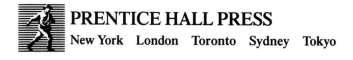
PRENTICE HALL PRESS
New York   London   Toronto   Sydney   Tokyo

Published in 1987 by Prentice Hall Press
A Division of Simon & Schuster, Inc.
Gulf + Western Building
One Gulf + Western Plaza
New York, New York 10023

This is a revised edition of a work originally published by the American Diabetes Association® under the title *Learning about Diabetes*.

PRENTICE HALL PRESS is a trademark of Simon & Schuster, Inc.

Library of Congress Cataloging-in-Publication Data

Diabetes in the family, rev. ed.

Bibliography: p.
Includes index.
1. Diabetes—Popular works. I. American
Diabetes Association. [DNLM: 1. Diabetes
Mellitus—popular works.   WK 850 D536]
RC660.D449   1986   616.4′62   86-25384
ISBN 0-13-208653-0

Designed by Stanley S. Drate/Folio Graphics Co. Inc.

Manufactured in the United States of America

10 9 8 7 6 5 4 3 2

ACKNOWLEDGMENTS

I wish to thank Oscar B. Crofford, M.D., President of the American Diabetes Association; Irving L. Spratt, M.D., President-Elect; Florence R. Ruhland, R.N., Vice President Health Professional; Boyd E. Metzger, M.D., Chairman of the Education Division; John W. Runyan, Jr., M.D., Chairman of the Committee on Patient Education; Charles M. Clark, Jr., M.D., Chairman of the Committee on Government Relations; Robert B. Zagoria, Esq., and Barbara El-Beheri, R.D., Nutrition Program Coordinator, for their patience, suggestions, and careful review of the manuscript. My thanks also to Marion Franz, R.D., and Judith Wylie-Rosett, R.D., for their help with the Basic Meal Plan and to Sally Burbee, Consultant, Health/Patient Education, for her painstaking editorial assistance.

For the encouragement and support of my coworkers on the ADA staff, Robert Bolan, Caroline Stevens, Amy Danzig, Robert S. Dinsmoor, and Ricki Rusting, I am most grateful. A special word of thanks to Myra Perry, my secretary, who diligently proofread much of the manuscript.

My appreciation goes also to those who contributed their expertise to the 1987 edition: R. Keith Campbell, R.Ph., Pasquale Palumbo, M.D., and Madelyn L. Wheeler, R.D., M.S.

To all of the people with whom I have talked and corresponded over the years, I am particularly indebted. You asked the questions about diabetes that made this book possible.

DOROTHY M. BORN
1982

CONTENTS

Preface   xi

Introduction   xiii

1 DIABETES THEN AND NOW   1

2 WHAT IS DIABETES?   7
What Kinds of Diabetes Are There?   8
Who Gets Diabetes and Why?   10
Do I Really Have Diabetes?   12
Controlling Diabetes   13
Adjustment to Diabetes   18
You Are in Charge   21

3 DIABETES DAY BY DAY   22
The Importance of Diet   22
What Is an Exchange?   26
Blood Tests   29
Urine Tests   33
Stress and Emotions   36
Exercise   39
Care for Your Feet   45
Keep Smiling   48
Skin Problems   51
When You Are Sick   53

4 LIFETIME CONSIDERATIONS   57
Alcohol   57
Smoking   59
Driving   60
Careers and Employment   61
Insurance   65
Travel   67
Marriage and Pregnancy   73

5 TYPE I, INSULIN-DEPENDENT DIABETES — 77
Goals of Treatment — 77
Insulin — 79
Insulin Injection Techniques — 84
Self-Management — 94

6 EMERGENCIES—BE PREPARED — 96
Insulin/Hypoglycemic Reactions — 96
The Somogyi Effect — 107
Ketoacidosis/Diabetic Coma — 108
Hyperosmolar Nonketotic Coma — 111

7 TYPE II—NON-INSULIN-DEPENDENT DIABETES — 113
Goals of Treatment (Weight Loss) — 113
What Is Obesity? — 114
The Diet Prescription — 116
Exercise and Weight Control — 119
Oral Drugs — 119
Interaction with Other Drugs — 120

8 PROBLEMS—COMPLICATIONS — 122
Blood Vessel Disease — 122
Visual Problems — 127
Kidney Disease — 131
Disease of the Nerves: Neuropathy — 134

9 DIABETES AND THE FAMILY — 138
Psychosocial Issues — 138
Resolving Conflicts — 139
Counseling — 140

10 DIABETES IN LIFE STAGES — 144

11 THE PROMISE OF RESEARCH — 151
Genetics and Immunology — 152
Transplants — 152
Implantable Glucose Sensor/Pump — 153
Nutrition — 154
Insulin Resistance — 155
Obesity — 155

12 RESOURCES 157

A Basic Meal Plan 157
Exchange Lists for Meal Planning 159
Publications of the American Diabetes Association 173
The American Diabetes Association Affiliates 174

Bibliography 179

Glossary of Medical Terms 181

Index 185

PREFACE

If you have diabetes you belong to a very large and growing family. There are more than 11 million of you in the United States today. Some of you are children and young adults; many of you are middle-aged and older. You live in big cities, small towns, and in rural areas; you work in a variety of occupations. We know many of you through your letters, which over the years have poured into our offices all across the country by the tens of thousands. We know those first fears when diabetes is discovered, we share your frustrations in the day-to-day living with diabetes, and we feel your concerns for the future. Some of you have written to us of your successes and triumphs in living and dealing with this complex disease. Your stories have inspired others and encouraged us in our pursuit of knowledge about diabetes. In the words of the poet, "No man is an island . . .," and never is this more true than when diabetes strikes. Diabetes *afflicts* one member; it *affects* the whole family.

This book reflects your questions, your concerns, and your hopes for the future. We want to improve the quality of your life by providing you with accurate, useful, and up-to-date information. The book is divided into chapters starting with "Then and Now," a short history to show you how far we've come in the treatment of diabetes. The next chapter, "What Is Diabetes?" deals with the nature of diabetes and one's adjustment to it. Under "Day by Day" you will find general information on diet, blood and urine testing, exercise, stress, and foot, dental, and skin care. "Lifetime Considerations" covers questions about alcohol, smoking, driving, careers and employment, travel, insurance, marriage, and pregnancy. For quick reference there are separate chapters on the two types of diabetes. Other chapters include "Emergencies—Be Prepared," "Problems—Complications," "Diabetes and the Family," "Diabetes in Life Stages," and "The Promise of Research," which discusses current research. The final chapter lists resources for people with diabetes and their families. There is much to be learned about diabetes, but no one book will tell you all you need to know. We've tried to give you basic information to get you started.

The American Diabetes Association is as eager to find a preventive and a cure for diabetes as you are. While there has been a virtual explosion in knowledge and research since the passage of the National Diabetes Mellitus Research and Education Act of 1974, not all the questions have been answered. Until a cure is found, we feel it is our responsibility to you, our growing family, to teach you how to live a full and healthy life with diabetes. This is our job, and this is what this book is all about. You can live with diabetes. We can teach you how.

DOROTHY M. BORN

INTRODUCTION

In the past 10 to 20 years more progress has been made in the understanding of diabetes than in the previous half century. While it was thought at the time of the discovery of insulin in 1921 that the problems of diabetes were largely solved, it has become apparent that this is not the case. This book will present much current information about the problems of diabetes, its treatment, and its complications, in a style that most people will understand and appreciate. If you or a member of your family have recently been diagnosed as having diabetes, you have taken an important step in a long and useful life by seeking information about your condition. Review often the chapters and sections that are particularly relevant to your circumstances. Those of you with long-established diabetes will benefit by being brought up to date on the great progress made in all aspects of diabetes.

You will want to keep abreast of these advances in diabetes, and the American Diabetes Association, its affiliates, and chapters are prepared to help you. However, you must make them aware of your interest and needs.

This book is largely the work of Dorothy Born, who assembled the original manuscript in record time. She also played a key role in preparing the revisions for the 1987 edition. We all owe her our thanks for this great effort.

DANIEL PORTE, JR., M.D.
President
American Diabetes Association
1986–1987

Diabetes

IN THE

Family

Revised Edition

1

DIABETES THEN AND NOW

When you first learn that you have diabetes it may help to know that you are not alone. It is estimated that five hundred thousand new cases of diabetes are diagnosed every year and that there are more than 11 million people with diabetes in the United States today; unfortunately, almost half of them do not know they have the disease. Projecting figures still further, it now appears that if the incidence (new cases) of diabetes continues at the present rate, an American born today and living an average life span of 70 years has a one-in-five chance of developing diabetes, unless a cure or preventive is found. This increase in numbers is alarming. To researchers, and to all those concerned with the care and treatment of diabetes, the challenge to find the answers to the causes and cure is urgent.

Diabetes is not a new disease. Prescriptions to relieve thirst were recorded as early as 1500 B.C. Aretaeus, a Greek physician, was the first to identify diabetes and give it its name. In the second century A.D. he described diabetes as, ". . . a wonderful affliction not very frequent among men, being a melting down of the flesh and limbs into urine." The full name, diabetes mellitus, was given to the disease later. It comes from the Greek and Latin words meaning "to pass through" and "honey," describing the major symptom, sugar in the urine.

Maimonides, a twelfth-century physician, thought that diabetes was a disease of hot climates because he saw it frequently in Egypt but never in Spain. And Paracelsus, the most famous physician of the fifteenth century, thought that salt was the culprit. It wasn't until 1700, when Matthew Dobson demonstrated that the urine of a diabetic actually contained sugar, that the true nature of the disease was known. He proved this by tasting the urine.

Although little was known about nutrition in the early 1800s, many attempts to treat diabetes with diet were tried. Rollo, Naunyn, and Cantani were all advocates of a severely restricted carbohydrate diet, high in fat and protein. Their methods of getting patients to follow the diet ranged from one or more days of forced fasting per week, to locked-door confinement for those who did not comply. So distasteful was the diet in some cases that the patient preferred the disease to the treatment.

It had long been suspected that there was a connection between diabetes and the pancreas. In 1869 the body's insulin source, tiny clumps of insulin-producing cells in the pancreas, was identified by Langerhans. These cells were subsequently named the islets of Langerhans in honor of their discoverer. The relationship between diabetes and pancreas was proved conclusively in 1889 when the scientists von Mering and Minkowski produced diabetes in dogs by removing the pancreas. Today research scientists are trying to find ways to regenerate these cells by implanting healthy new islet cells (see chapter 11).

In the early 1900s Dr. Frederick M. Allen noticed in his experiments that when a part of the pancreas was removed, the remaining islet cells degenerated and diabetes developed. This led him to believe that the cells were being overworked, and he concluded that by resting the cells periodically they would rejuvenate themselves. To accomplish this he introduced a diet that alternated days of very meager nourishment with days of total fasting. Although this treatment kept the patient alive, it did not provide him with much energy.

Then in 1921, life for people with diabetes was radically improved by the discovery of insulin by Drs. Banting and Best. Prior to this time a diabetic person lived only a few years after developing the disease. In 1921 the first dose of insulin was given to a young man with diabetes, and his condition improved dramatically. In 1923 the commercial production of insulin was begun in the United States, and insulin became available for all persons with diabetes.

But the story does not end here. For a while it was thought that insulin was the whole answer to diabetes and that by injecting the missing hormone (a chemical substance produced in the body that circulates in body fluids and produces a specific effect on body cells), diabetes would be cured. Insulin did prolong life, but as it did it became apparent that patients were showing evidence of vascular (blood vessel) disease at an earlier age than was found in the general population. Scientists began to look further for improved methods of treatment. The first insulins were so short-acting that four injections a day were required. By contrast, insulins such as NPH and Lente, which are used now, start to lower blood sugar within an hour or two after injection, with the effect lasting up to twenty-four hours. These long-acting insulins only had to be given once a day, and it was thought that they would improve diabetes control by their extended effects. Their appeal, particularly for children, was enormous because they reduced the number of daily injections required.

In 1940 a group of physicians concerned with the increasing incidence of diabetes in the United States formed a professional society known as the American Diabetes Association (ADA). Their purpose was fourfold: to create better understanding of diabetes among patients; to promote the free exchange of knowledge and standards of treatment among physicians; to disseminate accurate information on the early recognition and need for medical supervision to the general public; and to promote research into the causes and the possible cure for diabetes. By the mid-1960s diabetes had become a major health problem, and the American Diabetes Association was reorganized as a voluntary health agency. With affiliates from coast to coast, the ADA today serves the interests of all people with diabetes and their families. Its programs in patient and professional education and its commitment to research are known the world over. The Association is in the forefront in bringing knowledge about diabetes to the public. These efforts culminated in the passage of the National Diabetes Research and Education Act of 1974, when for the first time in U.S. history, the federal government was committed to an investment of money for research in diabetes similar in scope to that being done in heart diseases, communicable diseases, and cancer.

In 1950 a revolution in the concept of diabetes was brought about by the research of Drs. Berson and Yalow, who developed a radioimmunoassay test (radioactive insulin traceable in the blood) that measures the amount of insulin in the blood. When the test was given to a group of diabetic persons, some of them showed evidence of normal and even high levels of insulin in their blood. Others showed no insulin at all. Up to this time it was thought that diabetes was caused by a lack of insulin. Now it became clear that there was another type of diabetes in which insulin effectiveness, not a lack of insulin, was the problem. Insulin resistance and the riddle of "maturity-onset" diabetes began to unfold.

In 1948 a group of scientists working with sulfa drugs discovered quite by accident that these drugs brought about hypoglycemia (lower than normal blood sugar) in animals. This discovery led to the development of the oral hypoglycemic compounds: drugs in pill form that stimulate the release of insulin by the pancreas. These drugs, while related to the sulfa drugs, are not effective against infection, but they have proved effective for short-term treatment in those diabetic people whose pancreases produce some insulin.

In 1950 the American Diabetes Association, in conjunction with the American Dietetic Association, published the first Exchange Lists, which greatly simplified the way in which people with diabetes could calculate their daily food intake. It had previously been necessary to weigh all the food eaten each day. Now it was possible to follow a prescribed daily meal plan by learning "exchanges," "trades," or "substitutions." The lists were revised in 1976 to reflect new knowledge about dietary fat and its relation to blood vessel diseases, and again in 1986 to reflect recent findings about the effects of sodium and fiber in the diet.

In 1959 the American Diabetes Association published *A Cookbook for Diabetics,* one of the first cookbooks written exclusively for the person with diabetes. Close to a million copies were purchased.

In 1971, 1979, and again in 1986, the Association affirmed its position that the diabetic person has essentially the same nutritional needs as everyone else. Daily diet is an individual consideration and should be prescribed to meet the physical and cultural needs of the person with diabetes. The nutritional goals of the diet are to achieve and maintain desirable body weight, to maintain blood glucose as close to normal as possible, and to prevent or delay the complications associated with diabetes insofar as they are related to diet.

In the fall of 1980 the Association authored the *Family Cookbook* in collaboration with The American Dietetic Association. The book is a guide to good eating for the whole family and includes much current knowledge of nutrition. A companion volume to the *Family Cookbook* was published in 1984, with 200 additional recipes. In 1986 the *American Diabetes Association Holiday Cookbook* was published, with more than 175 recipes geared to traditional American holidays.

During the last ten years much attention has been focused on the role of exercise in diabetes and its value in lowering blood sugar and preventing blood vessel disease. In 1979 the American Diabetes Association sponsored a Symposium on Diabetes and Exercise to study the benefits of exercise and its long-term effect on diabetes. As a result of the Conference, the ADA appointed an ad hoc committee on exercise and diabetes to identify areas in which information is lacking, to define the potential value of exercise to diabetes, and to establish guidelines for the individual exercise prescription.

In 1987 the Association established a Council on Exercise to provide a forum for professional members interested in the benefits, risks, and practical problems of physical exercise by people with diabetes. The council also disseminates information on the effects of exercise and strives to foster greater research interest in this area.

There is much new hope for people with diabetes today. Our knowledge about the disease has come a long way from starvation diets and prescriptions to relieve thirst. We don't have all the answers yet, but it is certain that the diabetic person today has a greater chance of living a longer and better life than was possible 25 or 50 years ago.

2

WHAT IS DIABETES?

Have you ever thought about what goes on in your body when you get out of bed in the morning, reach for a cup of coffee, or sprint out the door a little late for school or work? We know that energy speeds us on our way, but where does this energy come from?

The human body is made up of millions of tiny cells that need energy to work properly. These cells get the energy they need from the food we eat. Food is changed during digestion into the many chemicals essential for life, including a form of sugar called *glucose*. Some glucose is used for energy right away and some is stored for future used in the liver and in the muscles in the form of *glycogen*.

The pancreas, a large gland behind the stomach, produces several substances important in body processes. Two of these substances are hormones essential to energy production: *Glucagon*, produced by the alpha cells of the pancreas, helps to raise the blood sugar level by taking glycogen (stored glucose) out of the body reserves. *Insulin*, produced by the beta cells of the pancreas, help to lower blood sugar by transporting glucose from the blood into the cells. Normally, the pancreas automatically releases just enough of these hormones to keep the amount of blood glucose in balance at all times. This happens regardless of what food is eaten or what physical activity is undertaken, because if no glucose is readily available, the reserves of stored glycogen can be converted into glucose for use as energy.

For the cells to use glucose properly, insulin must be present. Insulin is the key that opens the cell door so that the glucose can enter. The process by which food is digested and chemically changed into glucose, the cells' energy source, is a continuous chain of events, each one dependent upon the other to produce energy. Everyone has glucose circulating in the blood at all times, but not everyone has sufficient or effective insulin. This then is diabetes.

In diabetes, the chain of events that produces energy is broken at the point where glucose normally enters the cells, either because of a total lack of insulin or because the insulin cannot be used effectively. When glucose cannot enter the cells it accumulates in the blood, is passed through the kidneys, and overflows into the urine, causing one of the classic symptoms of diabetes, frequent urination. When diabetes is untreated, as blood sugar rises and more and more glucose is lost in the urine, other symptoms such as extreme thirst, blurred vision, weakness, and weight loss occur.

Diabetes is the name for a group of chronic (lifelong) diseases that cannot as yet be cured but that can be controlled. It affects the way in which the body uses food.

WHAT KINDS OF DIABETES ARE THERE?

Type I, insulin-dependent diabetes, is sometimes called juvenile-onset diabetes because it usually occurs in children, adolescents, and young adults, although it can occur at any age. People with this type of diabetes produce so little insulin that daily injections are always necessary. The appearance of insulin-dependent diabetes is usually sudden and often severe. When insulin production stops abruptly, which happens in this type of diabetes, large amounts of sugar are trapped in the blood. The body is unable to move the glucose into the cells because of a lack of insulin and has to use its reserves of fat for energy. As this occurs, the body literally begins to feed upon itself, causing extreme weakness. Other symptoms include excessive thirst, frequent urination, irritability, nausea, hunger, and weight loss in spite of large amounts of food eaten. This type of diabetes is the more serious of the two main types and requires daily injections of insulin, a prescribed diet, and exercise in order to achieve control. It is estimated that insulin-dependent diabetes makes up about 10 percent of all cases.

Type II, non-insulin-dependent diabetes, is sometimes known as adult- or maturity-onset diabetes because it usually develops in persons over 40 years of age. Ninety percent of all people with diabetes are in this category. In Type II diabetes the pancreas produces some insulin, but it is either not sufficient for normal energy production or it cannot be used effectively. The symptoms include any of those for Type I diabetes, as well as the slow healing of cuts, fatigue, blurred vision, cramps in the legs, feet, and fingers, itching, and drowsiness. Many times the symptoms are so obscure that people don't discover they have diabetes until a routine medical examination reveals it. Eighty percent of those with non-insulin-dependent diabetes are overweight at the time of diagnosis. Often this type of diabetes can be controlled merely by bringing the weight down to normal and maintaining the loss. Some people in this category are given an oral drug or insulin, in addition to diet, to achieve control.

There is a subtype of non-insulin-dependent diabetes that occurs in people who are not overweight. About 10 percent of those with Type II diabetes belong to this group.

Gestational diabetes occurs during pregnancy. Women who develop it are tested and reevaluated after pregnancy, when blood glucose usually returns to normal. However 30 to 40 percent of such women will develop diabetes within 5 to 10 years.

Impaired glucose tolerance refers to a condition in which the fasting plasma glucose level (determined by a test performed after an overnight fast) is between normal and diabetic levels. The term replaces the terms borderline, chemical, or latent diabetes, which were formerly used. When this condition is found it is corrected with an appropriate diet, weight loss if necessary, and exercise to prevent it from developing into actual diabetes.

Secondary diabetes is associated with certain conditions or syndromes (a pattern of symptoms occurring together), such as diabetes induced by drugs or chemicals, pancreatic or endocrine disease. (The endocrine system is made up of the pancreas, thyroid, adrenal, pituitary, and gonad glands. These glands release chemical substances into the blood that regulate and control the various functions of the body.)

WHO GETS DIABETES AND WHY?

Heredity plays an important part in determining who gets diabetes; however, there is no clear pattern of inheritance, and no exact predictions can be made as to how the disease will appear in future generations. Parents of a diabetic child often wonder how their child could possibly have developed diabetes, when there is no history of it on either side of the family. This is a puzzling question, but we don't always know the medical histories of all of our ancestors. It may be that somewhere in the family tree diabetes did appear but may have gone undiagnosed.

It has been observed that insulin-dependent diabetes sometimes follows a viral infection such as mumps or Coxsackie. This indicates that disorders of the body's immune system (the system that helps to overcome infection and disease) may be responsible for triggering diabetes. Why do these viruses attack and destroy the pancreatic beta cells in some individuals and not in others? If an answer to this question could be found, then a vaccine to prevent diabetes would become a definite possibility.

Stress is another factor in the development of diabetes. Many diabetes specialists see the growth spurts during childhood, preadolescence, and puberty as a stimulus for diabetes in the genetically prone (those with the diabetic trait).

In non-insulin-dependent diabetes obesity is the single most important cause. As one doctor put it very bluntly, "If you want to avoid diabetes, don't get fat." Where there is a family history of obesity and diabetes, if one family member is overweight and another is not, the obese member is more likely to develop diabetes.

Non-insulin-dependent diabetes may also be unmasked by stress, either physical or emotional, such as a serious illness or accident, the death of a spouse, divorce, or the loss of a job. It is not uncommon for a person in the middle years to be admitted to the hospital for a heart attack, stroke, or some other condition, only to learn that he/she also has diabetes.

The stress of pregnancy can trigger diabetes too. This is particularly true of women who have a history of having borne larger than average-size babies.

Summary: The factors that contribute to the onset of diabetes are thought to be heredity, viral infections, obesity, severe stress, and pregnancy.

Why is diabetes increasing at such an alarming rate? Statistics reveal that diabetes affects 11 million Americans directly and an estimated 50 million indirectly. It appears that diabetes is on the increase today because people are living longer than ever before in history, and the chance of developing diabetes increases with each decade of life after 40 years of age.

Our environment is probably another reason for this increase. We are eating more and exercising less. The farmer no longer walks behind his plow or threshes his wheat by hand; machines do it for him. In our towns and cities, we ride to work in cars and buses and are carried to our offices by elevators. In the home, energy-saving devices have taken most of the physical labor out of housework. The stress of crowded city living, the lack of vigorous physical exercise, and the constant competition in the workaday world all multiply our chances for developing diabetes.

This theory of inactivity and high incidence of diabetes has been demonstrated by the late Kelly West in his studies among the Indian tribes of Oklahoma. He found that all the full-blooded Indians in the tribe over age 35 were overweight, and that one half of them had diabetes. Before 1940 diabetes was virtually unknown in the tribe. When the Indians began to migrate to the cities to find work, the stressful but sedentary life gradually replaced the active life they had known on the reservation. Their eating habits changed radically. Diets rich in processed food and high in calories, combined with a lack of exercise, led to a gradual and steady weight gain. Over a period of years this added weight placed more demands on the beta cells to produce more insulin. Eventually, the cells slowed down or even stopped producing insulin altogether. This appears to account for today's high incidence of diabetes in the tribe.

More recently a study of the prevalence of diabetes (total number of cases) in rural and urban Polynesian populations of Western Samoa showed that diabetes occurred almost three times more often in urban than in rural populations. The study suggests that a combination of factors—obesity, physical inactivity, and stress—may have contributed to this increased incidence.

Summary: In the light of our present knowledge, Type I diabetes cannot be prevented. The best way to prevent the development of Type II diabetes is to avoid obesity, particularly if there is a family history of diabetes.

DO I REALLY HAVE DIABETES?

Like thousands before you, when confronted with diabetes you probably wondered, do I, or does my child really have diabetes? How does the doctor know? The signs and symptoms may have provided some clues; for example, a blood or urine test high in sugar. Diabetes in children and young adults usually appears suddenly, and the symptoms are easily recognized. Often, however, the symptoms in older people are vague. In order to be sure, the doctor will order a blood test. It may be a test before breakfast or two hours after a meal. If blood glucose levels above normal limits are found, no further tests may be necessary. If there is any doubt, however, a "blood glucose tolerance" test may be given. This test shows how the body responds to a large amount of sugar in the blood.

The blood glucose tolerance test is given after an overnight fast (no eating for eight hours or more). The first sample—called a *fasting sample*—is then drawn. An amount of glucose based on height and weight is given either by injection or by mouth. Blood samples are drawn at one-, two-, and three-hour intervals. From these the doctor will chart your blood glucose curve to see how your body handles sugar. Figure 2–1 shows the test curves of three people: A has a normal curve and is not diabetic; B has impaired glucose tolerance; and C is diabetic.

Don't be confused by test numbers. Your reading may not compare with that of a friend. Testing methods vary. Blood glucose is measured in whole blood, serum, or plasma. Whole blood is blood as it comes from the vein. Serum or plasma is the fluid part of the blood in which cells are suspended. Your doctor will interpret the results according to the test he has ordered for you.

What Is a Normal Reading?

Many people ask, "What is a normal blood glucose level?" This is a difficult question to answer because what is normal for a child would not be for an adult. Many factors must be considered in reading the test results: age, physical condition, recent or current medication, illness, and infection. Only your doctor can determine what is normal for you.

CONTROLLING DIABETES

Good control of diabetes means keeping blood glucose levels as near to normal as possible.

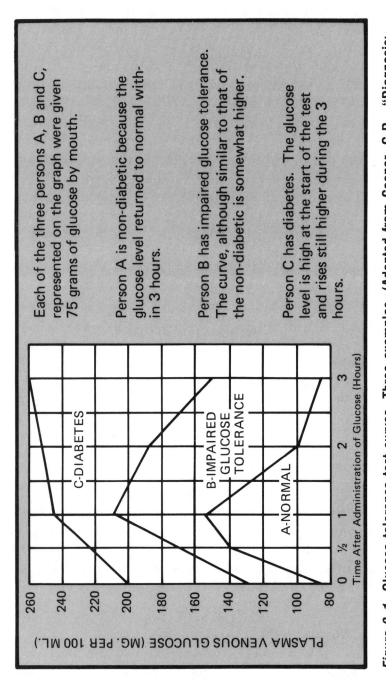

Each of the three persons A, B and C, represented on the graph were given 75 grams of glucose by mouth.

Person A is non-diabetic because the glucose level returned to normal within 3 hours.

Person B has impaired glucose tolerance. The curve, although similar to that of the non-diabetic is somewhat higher.

Person C has diabetes. The glucose level is high at the start of the test and rises still higher during the 3 hours.

Figure 2–1. Glucose tolerance test curves. Three examples. (Adapted from Cooper, G.R., "Diagnosis: Diabetes," *Diabetes Forecast* 33 [2]: 1980)

When you see someone on a skate board zigzagging gracefully down the street, you can be sure he's spent some hours practicing. It looks so easy, but actually it takes balance, control, and practice. Good control of diabetes is somewhat like riding a skateboard; it requires a balance of diet, exercise, and sometimes insulin or oral drugs, and it takes some practice too. In keeping this delicate balance, the person with diabetes does for himself what nature does automatically for the nondiabetic person. Good control requires a knowledge of your body's needs and practice in coordinating your daily schedule of meals, activity, and medication.

Much emphasis is placed on good control because studies have shown that elevated blood glucose over a period of time can cause blood vessel and other diseases, which can lead to complicatons in the eyes, kidneys, and nerves.

The following charts give a picture of the blood glucose response to a meal in two different people, one without diabetes and one with diabetes.

In figure 2–2 (nondiabetic) we see the blood glucose first at the fasting level, then rising in response to a meal, and then returning to the original fasting level.

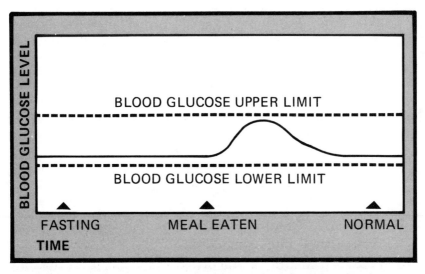

Figure 2–2. **Blood glucose response to a meal (nondiabetic).**

In figure 2–3 (untreated diabetic) the fasting blood glucose is above normal; it too rises after the meal but remains elevated.

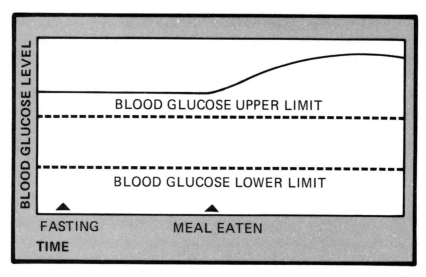

Figure 2–3. **Blood glucose response to a meal (untreated diabetic).**

In figure 2–4 the upper and lower limits of blood glucose are shown. When the upper limit of normal is passed, hyperglycemia (higher than normal blood suger) occurs, and when the level dips below the lower limit of normal, hypoglycemia (lower than normal blood sugar) is the result.

Your treatment goal should be to keep blood glucose as close to normal as possible. Your doctor will prescribe a course of treatment for you, depending on which type of diabetes you have. To help you in working toward good control, the following general guidelines are useful for all diabetics.

1. Keep your weight normal. Being overweight places stress on the entire body.
2. Take your insulin or oral drugs exactly as prescribed by your doctor.

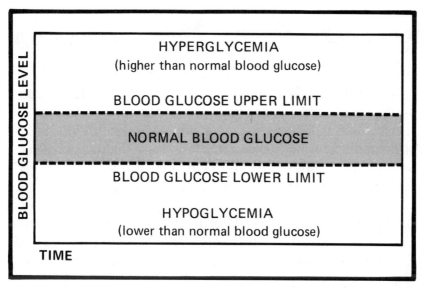

Figure 2–4. **Blood glucose response to a meal (treated diabetic).**

3. Take proper care of your eyes, teeth, skin, and feet. This is important because any infection can easily upset diabetes control.
4. Follow a regular program of exercise.
5. Don't smoke! Among other bad effects it constricts the blood vessels and impairs circulation.

Good control of diabetes has its own reward. You will feel good and look well. A young person with diabetes, poorly controlled for most of his life, was advised by his doctor to try two injections of insulin a day instead of one. He balked. He had always regarded his diabetes as a nuisance, and adding another injection to a daily schedule he already resented seemed like too much. However, his doctor finally persuaded him. Within six weeks he was a changed person. When he visited his doctor he appeared to be much healthier. He frankly admitted, "I never knew I could feel this good with diabetes. These days I feel as though I could lick the world."

ADJUSTMENT TO DIABETES

Good health is a blessing that we take pretty much for granted until it is threatened by illness or a chronic disease. If you have recently been diagnosed as having diabetes, or if you have had it for a while, you know the feelings of shock and disbelief you experienced when your doctor said, "You have diabetes." Many thoughts raced through your head: How will this affect my life? my family? my work? my plans? The news is shattering, whether it is given to the parents of a small child, to an adolescent with dreams for the future, or to a man or woman in the full stride of life. The onset may be gradual or it may be sudden, but it is always frightening (fig. 2–5).

To feel sorrow and a sense of loss is natural. It is natural to feel anger too. You are bound to ask yourself, "Why me? Why my child?" But the most difficult feeling to deal with is the sense of frustration. You are faced with a problem—diabetes—which you cannot solve and which you probably know very little about. It's like encountering an intruder in the dark; if he would just come out in the open you would know how to fight. You can't fight until you identify the enemy.

William Talbert, diabetic for more than 50 years, considers himself one of the lucky ones because insulin had just been discovered when he contracted diabetes. Treatment in the 1920s consisted of a carefully weighed diet, insulin injections, and a quiet life. But Bill had a loving and concerned father who decided that diabetes was not going to make an invalid of his son. He encouraged him to start playing tennis. Exercise was unheard of therapy for diabetes in those days. Within 4 months Bill had become the tenth-ranked young tennis player in the United States. He went on to become a national champion, was inducted into the International Tennis Hall of Fame, and still plays tennis regularly today.

Or take the case of Bill Gullickson, rookie pitcher for the Montreal Expos. He was stricken with diabetes just as spring

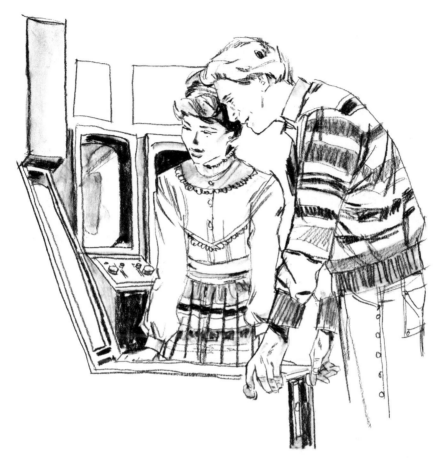

Figure 2–5. "Everyone has a problem. Mine is diabetes, but it doesn't stop me from enjoying life."

training was about to start. Back in high school he had promised himself a place in the major leagues by his twenty-first birthday. Now diabetes was threatening his big chance. He admits to being angry and scared at first. Then he remembered that Ron Santo, Catfish Hunter, and Bobby Clarke all have diabetes. He figured if they could make it, so could he. Six months later, with hardly a break in stride, he went on to pitch in the Expo's winning game against the San Diego Padres.

Not everyone who has diabetes becomes a celebrity, but diabetes is no cause to become a recluse or invalid either. With few exceptions people who have diabetes can choose almost any career, perform any work, or participate in any activity as successfully as their nondiabetic counterparts.

But learning to live with diabetes successfully requires determination and self-discipline, and not infrequently, some changes in the way you live. Teenagers may have a particularly difficult time in coping with diabetes because this is the time in their lives when it is painful to be "different." Blood and urine tests, insulin injections, and saying "No" to a shake with the gang after school can make you feel very different. Parents of young children with diabetes have not only the perplexing problems of a growing child to cope with but those of diabetes control as well. The middle-aged and elderly find changing the habits of a lifetime difficult and often bewildering.

How You Live with Diabetes Depends upon Your Attitude

You have a chronic disease that cannot be cured but that can be controlled. These are hard facts to face. However, if you count your blessings you will realize that diabetes, unlike many chronic conditions, is not crippling and doesn't show. You can still work, play, travel, and live much the same as you did before diabetes developed.

Everyone has a vast store of inner resources (faith, hope, courage, and determination) with which to meet the crises of life. By exploring and developing these you may discover qualities about yourself of which you were unaware. Your family and friends won't change because you have diabetes. Sharing your concerns about it with them will lighten your burden and give them a chance to help and support you.

Learn all you can about diabetes and how it can be controlled. Read about it, attend education classes, join groups of the newly diagnosed, and above all ask questions of your doctor or other health professionals. Don't let nagging doubts worry you. As you learn, you may find that having diabetes has some surprising dividends. Many times parents have told us that having diabetes in the family has changed all their lives for the better. As a family they are much more aware and concerned about their health now. The whole family is benefiting from their diabetic member's program of exercise and good nutrition.

YOU ARE IN CHARGE

It is generally agreed by all those who treat diabetes that there is no other disease in which the patient has to take so much responsibility for his or her own care. All the instructions, all the education given by the physician or health professional will be of no avail unless you take charge of your diabetes yourself. There is a saying, "knowledge is power," and with diabetes, the more you know about it and how it affects your body, the better you will be able to take care of yourself. This knowledge will put you in charge of your diabetes, and the result will be good health and freedom from worry.

Learn all you can, and use this knowledge to adapt and change your life to accommodate your diabetes.

As you learn more and more, your anger and frustration will fade. You will still have diabetes, but your perception of it will be changed. A thorough knowledge of the disease will change fear of the unknown into facts you can handle. When this happens you will be ready to relate to the simple wisdom of 10-year-old Karen, who was overheard explaining diabetes to her best friend.

"Sure, I have diabetes and I have to take shots every day, but otherwise I'm O.K."

"Is it catching?" asked her little friend.

"No!"

"Can you still play?"

"Of course silly, it's just diabetes!"

3

DIABETES
DAY BY DAY

THE IMPORTANCE OF DIET

Diet is the cornerstone in diabetes treatment because as we learned earlier, diabetes affects the way the body uses food. Food is necessary to life and growth and to provide energy. It is the fuel that keeps the motor of the body running smoothly. But food has another purpose too; it satisfies hunger.

The breaking of bread is one of man's oldest customs; it is a symbol of friendship and sharing. When we meet an old friend or make a new one, before parting we frequently agree to meet again soon, probably for lunch or dinner. At the family table we gather to share our food and our lives with one another. Eating is necessary to life, it is pleasurable, and it gratifies both physical and social needs.

In order to stay healthy, everyone should have a well-balanced diet. Having diabetes is no barrier to the enjoyment of good food. However, the person with diabetes must plan to get the best possible nutritional value from his prescribed meals.

The foods we eat are made up of proteins, carbohydrates, fat, vitamins, minerals, and water. These substances are known as nutrients. Each nourishes the body in a different way; together they sustain life, promote growth, and keep the body healthy.

Protein comes from two sources: animal and plant. Proteins of animal origin are found in milk, meat, poultry, fish, eggs, and cheese. Proteins of plant origin are found in dried peas, beans, nuts, grains, and cereals. Protein is used by the body to repair, replace, and maintain tissue.

Carbohydrates are divided into two types: complex and simple. Complex carbohydrates are found in pasta, bread, cereal, rice, and vegetables. Simple carbohydrates are found in honey, syrup, candy, table sugar, jams and jellies, cakes, pastries, and sweetened beverages and desserts. Carbohydrates provide the body with quick energy.

Contrary to popular opinion, everyone benefits from some carbohydrate in the diet. However, people with diabetes must limit the amount of simple carbohydrates they ingest, because these are absorbed quickly and cause a rapid rise in blood sugar.

Fiber is found in some carbohydrate foods and comes from the part of plant food that is not completely digested. Fiber is found in whole grain breads and cereals, and in vegetables and fruits, especially when the skin and edible seeds are eaten. It provides a feeling of fullness which helps those watching their weight. It stimulates the digestive process and prevents constipation.

Fat is useful in the diet as a source of fatty acid—which cannot be produced in the body—as a carrier for the fat-soluble vitamins, A, D, E, and K, and as a reserve of body fuel. Fat is digested slowly and thereby provides a feeling of fullness. Fat comes from two sources: animal and plant.

Animal fat (saturated, and hard at room temperature) is found in such foods as beef, pork, lamb, butter, milk, and cheese. Fat of plant origin is found in some margarines, some salad and cooking oils, and nuts. This fat is polyunsaturated and is soft at room temperature. Fat found in olives, nuts, and oils is also derived from plants. It is monounsaturated and soft at room temperature.

Of all the nutrients, fat is the richest source of calories. It contains twice as many calories per gram as either protein or carbohydrate. It is more satisfying than either protein or carbohydrate because it takes longer to digest. Obviously, though, eating too much fat will add unwanted pounds and can cause excessive amounts of cholesterol in the blood.

Cholesterol is a pearly, fatlike substance found in animal fat and also produced in the human body. Foods high in cholesterol include egg yolks, organ meats, sardines, and shrimp. Saturated fats tend to raise blood cholesterol; polyunsaturated fats lower it, and monounsaturated fats neither raise nor lower blood cholesterol. Although it has not been conclusively proven, it is now thought that a high consumption of saturated fat contributes to atherosclerosis (a narrowing of the blood vessels due to deposits of cholesterol and other substances).

Vitamins are organic substances that are essential to good nutrition. They are found in many foods in small quantities. They contribute to normal growth and the healthy functioning of body processes. The main vitamins are A, D, E, B Complex, C, and K.

Minerals such as calcium, iron, magnesium, phosphorus, potassium, sodium, and zinc are essential substances found in small amounts in most foods. Minerals aid in bone formation and strength, help to repair body tissue, and contribute to the control of body processes.

Water is as important to the body as air. It is possible to live for weeks without food but only for a few days without water. The body gets water from food that is eaten and broken down in the digestive process, and from liquids.

Besides nourishing the body, food also supplies energy, which is measured in calories. A calorie is a unit of heat or energy produced by food. Almost every food contains calories, but some foods are higher in calories than others. For example, a gram of carbohydrate in food provides 4 calories; a gram of protein in food also has 4 calories; but a gram of fat in food provides 9 calories. The number of calories in a food is equal to the sum of the calories of carbohydrate, protein, and fat it contains. Below are some examples of familiar foods showing their carbohydrate, protein, fat, and caloric content:

	Carbohydrate (grams)	Protein (grams)	Fat (grams)	Calories
1 8-oz. glass of skim milk	12	8	trace	90
½ cup of string beans	5	2	0	25
1 apple	15	0	0	60
1 slice of bread	15	3	0	80
1 oz. of chicken	0	7	3	55
1 oz. of ground beef chuck	0	7	5	75
1 tsp. of margarine	0	0	5	45

While it is desirable that the daily diet include some of each of the nutrients, protein, carbohydrate, fat, vitamins, minerals, and water each day, it is very important that the total calories consumed be just sufficient to meet the daily needs of the body in order to avoid either obesity or weight loss.

In 1986 the American Diabetes Association issued an official policy statement, "Nutritional Recommendations and Principles for Individuals with Diabetes Mellitus," which said, "Calories should be prescribed to achieve and maintain a desirable body weight."

For people with Type I diabetes, in order to keep diabetes under good control, two things are necessary: (1) to properly time meals, snacks, and exercise in relation to the action of insulin; and (2) to maintain day-to-day consistency in the amount of carbohydrate, protein, and fat in the diet.

For overweight people with Type II diabetes, the most important consideration is restricting *total calories* to achieve weight loss. In people with Type II diabetes, some insulin is produced and is circulating in the blood for use as the body demands, and regularity of meals and activity will prevent undue demands on the available insulin. Further information on meal planning for each type of diabetes can be found in chapters 5 and 7, respectively.

The question of additional vitamins in the diet of people with diabetes often arises. If your diet includes a variety of foods you are probably getting enough vitamins and minerals. Supplements may be needed when calorie intake is lower than 1,200 or 1,000 calories. Your doctor will prescribe them if necessary.

Your meal plan is individual. It will be prescribed for you by your diet counselor or doctor. It will provide enough calories to meet your energy needs, according to your age, sex, size, and physical needs. It will include foods that you enjoy and find satisfying. Favorite family recipes can be incorporated into the diabetic meal plan and your diet counselor will show you how to do this. The American Diabetes Association recommends that 55 to 60 percent of total daily calories should come from carbohydrates, mainly complex carbohydrates, 12 to 20 percent from protein, and less than 30 percent from fat. The level of saturated fat should be less than 10 percent of the total calories, with polyunsaturated fats making up approximately 6 to 8 percent, and the remainder made up of monounsaturated fat. Your diet prescription will probably be calculated in exchanges, which will make it simple for you to follow.

WHAT IS AN EXCHANGE?

Some people find food exchanges puzzling at first, but they are really very easy to understand. Think of an "Exchange" as a "trade" or a "substitute." There are six Exchange Lists, (1) Starch/Bread, (2) Meat, (3) Vegetables, (4) Fruit, (5) Milk, and (6) Fat. See chapter 12 for complete lists. Any food in a given list may be traded (exchanged) for any other food in that list in the amounts stipulated. Here is how it works. For example, when choosing from the Fruit List you will see that a small apple is equal to a small orange or to any of the other forty fruits listed in the amount specified. The same is true of the Vegetable List; one half cup asparagus is equal to, and can be traded for, one half cup zucchini. Turning to the Meat List you will see that an ounce of very lean beef is equal to an ounce of fish. If your breakfast meal plan calls for 1 fruit, 2 bread, 1 meat, 1 milk, and 2 fat exchanges, it could be interpreted like this:

```
1 fruit   = 1 small sliced orange
2 bread   = 2 slices of whole wheat toast
1 meat    = 1 boiled egg
1 milk    = 1 8-oz. glass of skim milk
2 fat     = 2 tsp. margarine
```

Your meals need never to be dull; they can be just as appealing and appetizing as you care to make them. By using the Exchange Lists imaginatively you can vary your diet in endless combinations. Once you know your basic meal plan, have mastered the Exchange Lists, and can gauge an exchange of food with your eye, you can enjoy eating away from home.

Here are some tips to remember when eating in a restaurant or in the home of friends.

1. Know the foods included on each Exchange List.
2. Know the "Exchanges" in your own prescribed meal plan.
3. Become familiar with serving sizes. You can do this by practicing at home. Don't be afraid to leave food uneaten if it doesn't fit into your meal plan.
4. Don't hesitate to ask questions about how a food is prepared, if you have any doubt about its suitability for you.

Try to avoid the following foods: thick soups, sweetened fruit juices, fatty, fried, or creamed foods, gravies or sauces, salads served with dressing, and sweet desserts.

When dining at the home of a friend don't be ashamed to say "No" to a food that is not for you. Now that dieting has become a way of life for a variety of reasons, your hostess will understand without a lot of explanation on your part.

If you are insulin-dependent, when dining out and the dinner hour is uncertain, you can eat a portion of your meal such as a Bread Exchange before leaving home and omit it later at dinner. This will make you feel more comfortable should dinner be delayed beyond your usual hour.

The dietary goals for people with diabetes are:

- To improve overall health
- To attain and maintain ideal body weight
- To provide for adequate physical growth in children and for the growth of the fetus (baby) in pregnant women
- To keep blood glucose and blood fat levels as near to normal as possible
- To make the diet realistic and attractive
- To achieve consistency in timing of meals for people with Type I diabetes and weight management for obese people with Type II diabetes

Sugar Is Known by Many Names

Simple sugars are carbohydrates that are quickly absorbed into the blood stream, and for this reason their use by people with diabetes should be sharply limited. All sugars are nutritive, which means that they contain calories, and these calories must be counted. It is good to familiarize yourself with some names of the more common sugars that you are likely to see on labels.

1. Sucrose, or table sugar, derived from sugar beets and sugar cane and includes granulated, powdered, brown, and invert sugars
2. Corn sugar, made from cornstarch
3. Corn syrup, a combination of several sugars and cornstarch
4. Fructose, a sugar found naturally in honey, plants, and some fruits and berries, and produced commercially from cornstarch
5. Honey, a syrup derived from fructose
6. Lactose, a sugar found in milk
7. Mannitol, a sugar alcohol found in many plants
8. Sorbitol, a sugar alcohol found in some plants and vegetables
9. Xylitol, a sugar alcohol found in almost all plants

Fructose and sorbitol are calorie-containing sweeteners that do not cause a significant sudden rise in blood sugar in people with well-controlled diabetes. Discuss with your diet counselor or doctor how these can be incorporated in your diet for an occasional treat. The use of fructose and sorbitol is not recommended for people with diabetes who are on a weight-loss diet because they do add calories.

Saccharin, a nonnutritive sweetener, has no calories. The American Diabetes Association recommends that its use be limited in children, young people, and pregnant women.

Aspartame (Equal®, NutraSweet®) is a manmade sweetener made from aspartic acid and phenylalanine, two of the amino acids contained in proteins. It is digested in the body as protein. Although aspartame has the same calorie content as sugar, it is 200 times sweeter, and therefore a very small amount is needed to satisfy taste. Thus, the calories added to the diet when aspartame is used are insignificant, an important consideration for people who have diabetes. Aspartame is acceptable as a sugar substitute in the diabetic meal plan, provided it is not used in large amounts.

BLOOD TESTS

A Test that Can Be Done at Home

A few years ago only your doctor could perform a blood test. Now there is a test that you can do at home. Self-monitoring of blood glucose is one of the most important advances in diabetes treatment in the past 40 years. It has changed completely the way in which people manage their diabetes.

Why Should I Test My Blood?

Testing your blood gives you a "reading" on the amount of glucose in your blood at the moment of testing. Blood tests are more accurate than urine tests because they show the *exact* amount of glucose, whereas urine tests show only the *percentage* of glucose. When blood tests are performed regularly and correctly, and the results are recorded, you and your doctor can follow the course of your diabetes. People with diabetes can learn to control their blood glucose level by observing the times of day when blood glucose is high or low. Your doctor will teach you how to alter your diet or activity to bring the level as close to normal as possible. This is known as "tight control" and is desirable because recent studies indicate that keeping blood glucose as close to normal as possible at all times may delay or even prevent the complications of diabetes.

Who Should Self-Monitor Blood Glucose?

The American Diabetes Association recommends self-monitoring of blood glucose for people who use insulin (especially those with hard-to-control diabetes), pregnant women, insulin pump users, those prone to severe ketosis, those prone to severe hypoglycemia who may not experience the usual warning symptoms, and those with a high renal threshold (the point at which glucose spills over into the urine; see fig. 3–1). The test may also be useful for persons with Type II diabetes.

When Should You Test?

Testing four times a day is usually recommended for people with Type I diabetes: before breakfast, after meals, and at bedtime, and more often when prescribed by the doctor.

For people with Type II diabetes, two times a day after meals, or perhaps two or three times per week may be sufficient, depending upon the individual circumstances and the doctor's advice.

How Is the Test Performed?

Blood is taken from the finger tip with a lancet, a device designed to draw a single drop of blood. The blood is placed on a chemically treated strip, and depending upon the strip used, blotted after 30 or 60 seconds, and read after 60 to 90 seconds, either visually or with a meter. Your doctor will advise on the testing and reading methods best suited to your needs. It is important to receive training from your health-care team on the mechanics of testing and to check your technique periodically.

What Products Are Used in the Tests?

For visual reading the following strips are available: Chemstrips bG, Glucostix, TrendStrips, and Visidex II.

When using a meter, use the strip recommended by the meter manufacturer.

Meter	Strips
Accu-Chek II	Chemstrip bG
BetaScan	TrendStrips
BetaScan B	TrendStrips
Diagem	Chemstrip bG
Diascan	Diascan
Diatron Easy	Diatron Easy Test, Chemstrip bG, Dextrostix (wet wash method)
Glucochek SC	Chemstrip bG
Glucometer II	Glucostix
Glucoscan 2000	Glucoscan test strips
Glucoscan 3000	Glucoscan test strips
TrendsMeter	TrendStrips

Source: From *Diabetes Forecast* 39 (3): 1986.

What Should My Blood Glucose Level Be?

Blood glucose levels vary among individuals, but the following chart shows approximate levels for various times of the day:

Blood Glucose Levels	Normal mg/d1	Probably Acceptable
fasting (before breakfast)	60–110	120 or less
1 hour after eating	100–150	185 or less
2 hours after eating	90–150	165 or less
premeal/bedtime	80–130	150 or less

Source: From Diabetes '85 fall issue.

Getting the Answers

In any test it is important to get the right answers. To achieve the greatest benefit from your blood tests: (1) follow the directions on the product you use as to timing, blotting, reading, and recording, (2) apply enough blood to cover the chemically treated portion of the strip, (3) store strips according to the directions on the package, and (4) when purchasing a new supply, always check the expiration date.

Using the Results

Merely testing your blood and recording the results is not enough. You will need to learn how to act on the results. Your doctor will review your record with you at each visit, show you how to alter diet, activity, or insulin, and, if necessary, correct any errors in performing the test.

Renal Threshold

Glucose, a sugar in the urine (glycosuria), is related to the level of glucose in the blood during the time urine is collecting in the bladder. When the blood glucose exceeds the normal renal (kidney) threshold of approximately 150 to 200 milligrams, glucose appears in the urine. Renal threshold,

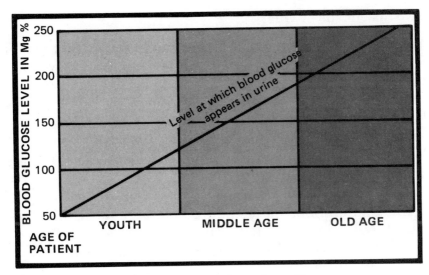

Figure 3–1. **Renal threshold normally varies with age.**
(From: *Diabetes Forecast* **31 [4]: 1978)**

the point at which glucose spills over into the urine, varies. Some people, particularly the very young, may have a low threshold, and sugar will appear even when blood glucose is not significantly elevated. In general, however, renal threshold rises with age. Some elderly patients may not spill sugar in their urine until the level in the blood is well over the 200-milligram mark (fig. 3–1).

URINE TESTS

As mentioned earlier, urine tests are not as *exact* as blood tests, but they do serve a useful purpose as an indicator of blood glucose control. They can be used alone to monitor glucose control, or they can be used as a supplement to blood glucose testing. As in blood testing, regularity, accuracy, and correct recording of the results will enable your doctor to follow your progress. From your record, he/she can make any necessary changes in treatment.

Two Specimens or One?

Your doctor will tell you whether he wants you to test the first or second morning urine samples, or both. You may think this is a nuisance, but there is a good reason for it. The first urine specimen reveals blood glucose levels over the past few hours; a second urine specimen shows control closer to the time of testing. For example, urine that has collected in the bladder overnight may show a higher glucose level than is actually present at the time of testing. The correct method of collecting second voided urine samples is to empty the bladder, take a drink of water, wait 20 to 30 minutes, and then take a second sample for testing. For those with Type II diabetes who run mostly negative tests, a second test is usually not necessary.

What Urine Tests Are There?

There are a variety of urine testing materials designed for specific use. Your doctor will tell you what materials to use. Following is a list of products available.

Chemstrip uG	strips, test for glucose only
Clinistix	strips, test for glucose only
Clinitest	tablet, tests for glucose only
Diastix	strips, test for glucose only
Tes-Tape	tape, tests for glucose only
Chemstrip uGK	strips, test for glucose and ketones
Keto-Diastix	strips, test for glucose and ketones
Kyotest UGK	strips, test for glucose and ketones
Acetest	tablet, tests for ketones only
Chemstrip uK	strips, test for ketones only
Ketostix	strips, test for ketones only

Source: From "Urine Testing Today." *Diabetes Forecast* 30(3): 1986.

Each product has a specific range and procedure for testing. Follow the instructions on the package insert.

Here are some tips for getting the most from your tests: test as soon as possible after voiding; do not expose strips, tablets, or tape to humidity, light, or heat; store at room temperature below 86°F, but do not refrigerate; never use after the expiration date or when a stick is bent or discolored.

Some factors that may affect accuracy and cause false positives or negatives are: exposure to chlorine or chlorine products, large doses of aspirin or vitamin C, and some antibiotics. Read carefully the package insert on the testing material you use so that you will be aware of these possibilities.

When Should You Test Your Urine?

People with Type I diabetes usually test before each meal and at bedtime. Tests at these times show how well your plan of food, activity, and insulin is working for you.

People with Type II diabetes usally test before one or more meals or after the principal meal of the day, because blood glucose is highest at that time. Your doctor will tell you when to test.

The sticks and tape can be used by Type II patients. These are not recommended for Type I patients for regular use because they do not indicate when large amounts of glucose are present. However, they can be used for convenience when traveling or at other times when necessary.

What Are Ketones and When Should You Test for Them?

When the body does not have enough insulin to release glucose for use in the cells, it starts to burn its own stores of fat. This causes tiny fragments of fatty acids, or ketones (sometimes called acetone, which is one form of ketone) to appear in the urine. Ketones usually appear at times of illness or infection. Three materials are used to test for ketones: Acetest, Chemstrip uK, and Ketostix strips. Perform the test according to the instructions on the package.

Summary: Both blood and urine tests give you a "reading" of your diabetes control. However, blood tests are more precise. Your doctor will review your record with you and show you how to monitor your own control.

Hemoglobin A₁C: The Blood Test that Looks Back

This is a test that reviews the pattern of your diabetes control. Research has shown that when blood glucose is elevated, it attaches to a chemical called hemoglobin, carried in the red blood cells as they circulate in the blood. This attachment is permanent and lasts for the life of the cell, which is approximately 120 days. When the amount of glucose that is bound to hemoglobin is measured, your doctor is able to see your pattern of control during the past three to four months. This information enables the doctor to alter your diet or insulin, if necessary, to achieve better control. The full name of the test is Glycosylated Hemoglobin A_1C. It is *not* a home test; it must be performed in the doctor's office. It does *not* replace the Blood Glucose Tolerance Test for the diagnosis of diabetes discussed earlier.

STRESS AND EMOTIONS

Stress and emotions can have an effect on your diabetes. There are two kinds of stress: that which is good and moves us to do our best in a challenging situation; and the stress that threatens us with danger or discomfort. We cannot avoid stress or eliminate it completely from our lives, nor would we want to. Just as spice added to food makes it tastier, stress adds zest to life. Without it our days would be dull and monotonous.

Webster defines stress as, "an outside force sufficient in strength to distort or deform." It is a demand made on the body and the mind by the environment, people, places, and things that requires us to alter our behavior. Stress can also be a threat or an expectation of future discomfort that puts us on alert. How we see stress, how we experience and cope with it, is our emotional response. Stress can be likened to the strong wind that fills the sails of a boat, and emotion to the skillful sailor who, by adjusting the sails, takes advantage of the wind and guides the boat in the direction he wants it to go.

Having a chronic disease is a stress in itself. When a group of people were asked what bothered them most about diabetes, they had many different answers, but all had a common thread, guilt.

"I didn't do what I was supposed to do."

"I really blew my diet this week."

"I don't check my urine every day. I know I should, but it's such a nuisance."

"I cancelled my regular appointment with my doctor because I knew my diabetes was out of control and I didn't want to face him."

These are all perfectly normal feelings, but they represent a denial of diabetes, and denial is stressful. These people haven't yet altered their sails to catch the wind. When stress is handled effectively it encourages us to overcome obstacles.

How Stress Affects the Body

When a sudden stressful situation develops, our nervous system responds to the threat of danger by signaling the pituitary and adrenal glands to secrete hormones. The released hormones cause the pupils of the eyes to enlarge, the hands and feet to perspire, the blood pressure to rise, and the heart rate to increase. Breathing becomes more rapid and more oxygen is needed by the lungs. Blood is diverted from the internal organs to the brain and body muscles, where it provides energy for thinking and acting in the threatening situation. This is the body's natural defense when faced with a threatening situation. At such times we experience the emotions of anger and fear.

So much for the sudden stress event. Suppose the threat is just as real but develops slowly over a period of days or weeks; anxiety builds, fear gnaws away inside. It may be some aspect of your diabetes that is worrying you, or a teacher, a boss, or a coworker who is giving you a difficult time and making you feel threatened. If you are a parent, perhaps a loveable, outgoing teenager has suddenly turned into a disagreeable stranger. It may be caused by the serious illness of a spouse or a close relative. Whatever the reason, the stress builds and builds. We have seen how many physical changes occur in the body as it prepares itself to cope and with sudden stress, but the slowly developing stressful situation can be just as damaging. Continuous stress keeps the body tense and anxious, in a state of combat readiness. This puts a strain on every organ. Diabetes may be one of the reasons for your stress, but when it is coupled with other stressful problems, your blood glucose control can be affected.

How Can You Reduce Stress in Your Life?

Look at the persons, places, or things that you find particularly stressful and try to change your thinking about them. Does something about your diabetes worry you? What bothers you the most? Answering these questions honestly will help you face your problem squarely. Then try talking it over with someone. Discussing your concerns with your physician, a health professional, a sympathetic friend, or a favorite family member will often give you a whole new outlook.

If you can't avoid a stressful life situation, try your best to alter it. If your boss is the problem, maybe you can find another job in a more congenial atmosphere. If this is unrealistic, try to change the way you see your problem so that your emotional response won't drain you of your energy and your zest for living. The way a person thinks creates the feelings of anger, anxiety, and frustration; it does not create the situations themselves.

The following is a list of tips for relieving stress.

- Identify the cause of your stress.
- Recognize the symptoms of stress as they build.
- Know your stress tolerance.
- Set aside 30 minutes a day for vigorous exercise if you are physically fit. An active body creates a calm mind.
- Learn relaxation techniques such as deep breathing exercises for relieving stress.
- Set aside a time each day for quiet meditation to relax the body and stretch the mind.
- Learn a new craft or skill. Spend some time each day on a favorite hobby.

Remember: Stress is only harmful when it becomes excessive. You will feel better, and your diabetes will be in better control, once you learn how to handle your stress.

EXERCISE

When man began to use his head instead of his feet, life became much easier, but a whole Pandora's box of diseases related to his new-found freedom was released; obesity, hypertension, arteriosclerosis, and diabetes, to name a few. Many of us go about our daily work without expending very much physical energy. A recent study revealed that $3 billion are lost annually to industry as a result of health problems. The study cited lack of stamina and little or no exercise as the principal reasons. Our huge sports arenas, filled to capacity every weekend, are testimony to the fact that we are a nation of enthusiastic spectators.

However, this picture is changing. The computer age has provided more time than ever before for leisure and recreation, and lately there seems to be an explosion of interest in exercise. More and more leisure hours are being devoted to jogging, skiing, swimming, tennis, handball, and a host of other sports. America, it seems, has awakened to the importance of physical fitness as a means of staying healthy (fig. 3–2).

When performed regularly, physical exercise is beneficial because it forces the muscles to work. It is especially good for people with diabetes because it lowers blood glucose by speeding the absorption of glucose in the cells. It improves circulation and muscle tone, contributes to weight loss in the obese, eases tension, and makes you feel good and look fit.

There is an exercise to suit every taste. There are the muscle-building ones like wrestling and weightlifting, and there are isometric exercises, which tighten muscles by tensing and relaxing techniques. There are contact sports, such as football, hockey, basketball, rugby, and soccer, which require teamwork and endurance. However, the best exercises for people with diabetes are those that are continuous and rhythmical, such as bicycling, walking, jogging, running, skating, swimming, cross-country skiing, and rowing. These are known as aerobic sports. Golf and tennis do not qualify as aerobic because they are "start and stop" sports and do not require sustained, continuous movement. These sports are not to be condemned, however, because any exercise carried out on a regular basis is beneficial.

The regular rhythm of aerobic exercise improves the flow of blood through the small blood vessels, increases the pumping power of the heart, and when done on a regular basis, slows the pulse rate. For people with diabetes who are prone to vascular disease, the benefits of aerobic exercise are a protection in warding off heart trouble and blood vessel disease.

In Type I diabetes exercise seems to enhance the action of injected insulin. As blood glucose is lowered, the body uses food more efficiently and little or no sugar (energy) is lost in the urine. Insulin-dependent people need to plan their exercise in accordance with their diet and the action of their insulin. Unplanned exercise or physical activity requires that an additional snack be eaten before beginning the activity, in order to avoid having too much insulin and too little glucose circulating in the blood, which would result in an insulin reac-

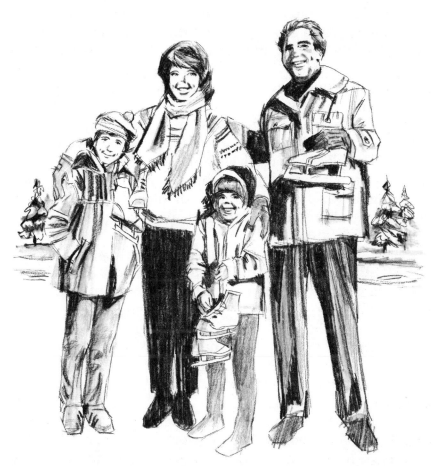

Figure 3–2. **Now the whole family is becoming more concerned about health.**

tion. An insulin or hypoglycemic reaction occurs when an excess of insulin causes the blood glucose to fall below 50 milligrams per 100 milliliters of blood. It is accompanied by sudden symptoms of trembling, sweating, and confusion; see chapter 6. Since insulin reaction related to exercise can be prevented by eating an additional snack beforehand, people with diabetes should always carry an extra snack of protein food, such as a sandwich or cheese and crackers, when exercise is anticipated.

Exercise is beneficial to insulin-dependent people if control is moderate to good. If control is poor, however, exercise can cause the blood glucose to rise. When undertaking a program of exercise, if your control has been poor, or if you are uncertain how good it has been, have your doctor examine you first.

If you are insulin-dependent, how you compensate for exercise is individual. For example, if you are a little overweight, your doctor may advise you to lower your insulin dose rather than eat extra food on the day you plan to exercise. How much you lower your dose should be discussed with your doctor after you have made some observations on how exercise affects you.

You can participate in unplanned activity by eating a snack before beginning. If a reaction develops while you are exercising, STOP, and take some form of carbohydrate that is quickly absorbed by the body. These include orange juice, sugar, or a nondiet soft drink. This will cause the blood sugar to rise and the symptoms of the reaction to disappear. It is important to remember that eating protein before the exercise will *prevent* low blood sugar. Carbohydrate (sugar) will *correct* low blood sugar.

Studies have shown that insulin injected in the leg is absorbed more rapidly when the leg muscles are used during exercise. This indicates that as blood circulation is increased by exercise, insulin gets to the cells faster. This suggests that when a sport using the legs in anticipated, insulin should be injected in either the arm or the abdomen.

People with Type II non-insulin-dependent diabetes who are overweight and underexercised should check with their doctor before starting any program of regular physical activity. People with this type of diabetes are not generally subject to hypoglycemic reactions. If you are over 40, your doctor may suggest a stress test (a treadmill test by which endurance is measured by pulse rate).

"Walking is man's best medicine." Hippocrates, the father of medicine, said this over 2,000 years ago. Although this advice went unheeded for a long time, for the person who has been living a sedentary life, walking is often the easiest way to start exercising. It can be done almost anywhere and at any time, and it requires no special equipment except comfortable shoes and proper clothing.

If you haven't exercised for a long time, inactivity has probably loosened some muscles and you look and feel heavier than you actually are, even though you may not be overweight. Regular exercise will help to tone the muscles. A sensible diet coupled with a program of regular exercise will help attain and maintain normal weight. A person who is physically fit can work longer and harder, and feel less tired, than someone who is not in good physical condition.

Beware of weekend exercise binges. Frequently they do more harm than good, and you will end up with sore muscles and few other noticeable benefits. Should bad weather or a tight schedule keep you from your daily walk or jog, you can always substitute indoor exercises for 10 to 15 minutes that day.

If you have been an armchair sport enthusiast, getting into the habit of regular exercise may hurt a bit at first, but the dividends are worth it. According to Dr. Fred Whitehouse, past president of the American Diabetes Association, and an enthusiastic advocate of exercise for people with diabetes, "The benefits of exercise go far beyond helping to control diabetes. Exercise has a tonic effect on the body. Your muscle tone improves; your sense of well-being and self-esteem grow. Your weight is easier to control; your step is lighter; your breath comes easier; general tension decreases."

The following are some things to remember as you start your program of exercise (they apply to both types of diabetes).

1. Whenever possible, exercise after a meal when blood glucose is rising.
2. Select an exercise or sport that you enjoy.
3. If you haven't exercised for a while, start slowly.
4. Exercise on a regular basis, daily if possible.

5. If you are insulin-dependent, adjust your food or insulin to accommodate your activity.
6. Wear good supporting shoes during exercise.
7. If you are overweight, remember that in order to lose one pound of fat you need to burn 3,500 calories; see table 3–1.

TABLE 3–1
EXERCISE AND CALORIES

Caloric Equivalents of Physical Exercise

2–2.5 cals/min	Light housework Strolling 1.0 mile/hr
2.5–4 cals/min	Level walking at 2.0 miles/hr Golf, using power cart
4–5 cals/min	Moderate housework, bowling, walking at 3.0 miles/hr Cycling at 6 miles/hr Golf—pulling cart Backpacking with light pack Dancing—modern, moderate
5–6 cals/min	Heavy housework or outside (yard) work, walking at 3.5 miles/hr (5.6 cal/min) Cycling 8 miles/hr Table tennis, badminton, and volleyball Golf—carrying clubs Tennis—doubles Many calisthenics and ballet exercises
6–7 cals/min	Walking 4 miles/hr Backpacking with heavy pack (40 lb—3 miles/hr) Cycling 10 miles/hr Ice or roller skating Basketball—half court Bowling Dancing—ballroom
7–8 cals/min	Walking 5 miles/hr Cycling 11 miles/hr Singles tennis

Source: Reprinted from the *Diabetic Athlete* with permission of the American Medical Association.

Note: This table represents the average number of calories expended for various forms of exercise. The actual calories expended may vary with the vigor of the exercise, but this table will provide a rough guide as to the number of calories that should be replaced. With diabetes, the "replacement" should preferably occur before the activity period to prevent causing the body to call upon its stores, thus increasing the risk of hypoglycemia if the stores are insufficient to meet the loss.

TABLE 3–1 *(continued)*

Caloric Equivalents of Physical Exercise

	Water skiing Dancing—square
8–10 cals/min	Jogging 5 miles/hr Cycling 12 miles/hr Downhill skiing, snowshoeing (2.5 miles/hr) Paddleball, soccer Swimming (recreational)
10–11 cals/min	Running 5.5 miles/hr Cycling 13 miles/hr Squash or handball

11–14 cals/min	Running—6 miles/hr
	         7 miles/hr
	         8 miles/hr
	Competitive swimming
	Judo, karate
	Football (while active)

14–20 cals/min	Wrestling Cross-country skiing Walking uphill 10–15% grade (3.5 miles/hr)
14–20 cals/min	Running at 7.5 miles/hr (15 cals/min) Running at 10 miles/hr (20 cals/min)

CARE FOR YOUR FEET

It is estimated that the average person walks three miles or approximately 20,000 steps each day. The twenty-eight small bones in each foot bear the full brunt of the body's weight with each step taken. They hold the body upright and keep it mobile, and yet this part of the human body often takes the most abuse. We seldom think of our feet until they hurt. Foot problems are not caused by diabetes, but when they occur in conjunction with it, they are more likely to be severe and develop quickly. This is particularly true if diabetes has affected the circulation and nerves (see chapter 8). Therefore, good foot care is of the utmost importance for the person who has diabetes.

Some common foot problems from which anyone can suffer are: cuts, scrapes, blisters, ingrown toenails, puncture wounds, athlete's foot, plantar warts, skin changes, mechanical problems involving the movement of bones and joints, and ulcers of the foot or leg.

Cuts, scrapes, and blisters can usually be treated at home with a mild antiseptic to avoid infection. Skin changes such as excessive dryness and itching can be relieved by daily careful bathing and the use of good skin creams. Every break in the skin of a diabetic person's foot must be viewed as serious.

You should seek prompt treatment by a professional when any of the following conditions appear.

- Ingrown toenails. These are easily recognized by redness, tenderness, and pain. Immediate treatment is necessary to avoid bacterial infection.
- Puncture wounds. These are always serious and should be treated promptly, as tetanus may be an added danger.
- Athlete's foot. This is a fungus infection; you may require a culture to determine the type of fungus so that appropriate treatment can be started.
- Plantar warts. These are encapsulated viral infections on the sole of the foot which are often very painful. They should receive prompt professional attention.
- Corns and calluses. These should be treated by a doctor or a podiatrist. Home surgery for these conditions is often the cause of serious and prolonged problems.
- Mechanical problems of the bones and joints, and deformities caused by poorly fitted shoes. These problems should receive professional attention.
- Ulcers of the foot will be discussed in more detail in chapter 8.

Foot Care Do's

1. Have your feet examined at least once or twice a year by a doctor or a podiatrist. Be sure to tell the doctor that you have diabetes.
2. Wash your feet daily, dry them well, and keep them dry. Always wear clean socks or stockings.

3. Inspect your feet daily, checking for redness, blisters, cuts, cracks between the toes, discolorations, or any other changes. Keep an eye on minor abrasions; keep them clean and treat only with antiseptics recommended by your doctor or podiatrist. If you notice any infection, changes, or abnormalities, report these immediately to your doctor. Because having diabetes may cause you to lose some feeling in your feet, regular foot inspection is essential. You could have an infection and not know it.

4. Prevent unnecessary cuts and irritations. Do not wear run-down shoes or worn-out stockings; do not treat your own foot problems with sharp instruments or by digging into the corners of the toenails; do not walk barefoot, even at home.

5. Avoid burns, including excessive sunburn. Do not put your feet in hot water or add hot water to a bath without testing the temperature. Generally, bath water should be between 85 and 90 degrees Fahrenheit. If you do not have a bath thermometer, test the water with your elbow. Avoid hot water bottles and heating pads. Check with your doctor regarding the use of an electric blanket on your bed.

6. Avoid doing things that restrict the blood flow to your feet, such as smoking, putting pressure on your legs, and exposing them to cold. (In a cold climate take precautions against frostbite.) Everyday activities that can put pressure on blood vessels in the legs and feet include sitting with the legs crossed and wearing round elastic garters or socks with tight elastic tops.

7. Do not use corn plasters or commercial corn cures. These contain preparations that are acidic and destroy tissue. Once you lose tissue, infection can easily develop.

8. When toenails are trimmed make sure they are cut or filed straight across, even with the top of the toe.

9. Always wear shoes that fit your feet and are suitable for the occasion. The widest part of the shoe should

match the widest part of your foot. The shoe should follow the natural outline of your foot and be snug but not too tight. Be sure to wear special shoes or have shoes specially made for your feet if you have a deformity.

In general, shoes should support the heel and keep your foot in position. There should be about three quarters of an inch of space beyond your longest toe when you stand. The toe box should be round and high to allow space for the toes to wriggle. The upper part of the shoe should be soft and flexible. Avoid wearing shoes made of plastic or other synthetic materials. These can cause your feet to sweat. Leather allows the feet to "breathe." The lining of the shoe should be smooth and free of ridges. Until you are used to new shoes, wear them for short periods and gradually lengthen the wearing time to accustom your feet to them.

10. If you have any type of foot infection, you need to test your urine and carefully monitor your blood glucose to determine the need for increased insulin.

KEEP SMILING

We are endowed with our teeth early in life. With careful and consistent care they should last a lifetime, which is what nature intended. Although no one is immune to dental problems, some problems seem to occur earlier and are often more severe in people with diabetes. (This does not apply to cavities, which are not more prevalent.) It is best to try to prevent problems before they occur.

Today periodontal disease is a common problem and is the cause of most tooth loss. The word comes from the Greek, peri "around" and odonto "teeth." It is a silent disease, and unlike a cavity, it causes no pain. It can develop as early as adolescence but not show itself until your 30s. Knowing how it develops and how it can be prevented will make you aware of the early symptoms and keep you brushing, flossing, and visiting your dentist regularly.

The teeth are held in place by the gums, the roots, and finally the jawbone. The gums surrounding the teeth are called *gingivae;* the bone that supports the root, the *cementum;* and the tissues that connect the roots to the jawbone, the *periodontal ligament* (fig. 3–3). Periodontal disease attacks all these structures, and if untreated destroys them systematically until the teeth become loosened and fall out.

Plaque, a film formed on the teeth by food, saliva, and bacteria, accumulates on the teeth, gums, and between the teeth. If it is not all removed by brushing, it hardens and turns into a substance called tartar. Bacteria, tartar, and plaque attack the gums and irritate them, causing them to become tender, swell, and bleed easily. This is the first stage of periodontal disease and is called gingivitis. As this progresses the poisons from the plaque gradually destroy the tissues that attach the teeth to the gums. The gums pull away from the teeth, creating pockets around them, and these become a source of infection. This is the second stage of periodontal disease and is known as pyorrhea. From this stage the disease progresses by weakening the supporting bones and loosening the teeth.

The first symptoms of periodontal disease are swollen, tender, and bleeding gums. Unfortunately, these symptoms do not appear early enough in the development of the disease to give a fair warning. But periodontal disease can be detected with X rays and a careful inspection by your dentist.

People with diabetes should be concerned about periodontal disease because it is usually more severe for them, and the destruction of the tissues and bones seem to happen more rapidly. This may be due to the fact that the small blood vessels that carry nutrients to the gums and the mouth become thickened, and circulation is slowed, setting the stage for infection. When diabetes is poorly controlled the hazards of bacterial infection are multiplied and the disease spreads even more rapidly.

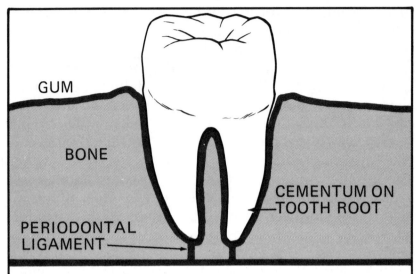

GUM

BONE

CEMENTUM ON
TOOTH ROOT

PERIODONTAL
LIGAMENT

The supporting structures of the teeth include: the gums surrounding the teeth, otherwise known as the gingivae; the cementum, the bone like outer covering of the tooth root; the periodontal ligament which connects the teeth to the sockets of the jawbone; and the jawbone itself.

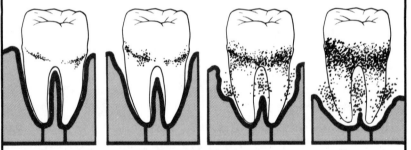

1. Plaque and calculus are deposited on teeth at gum line and cause gum irritation.
2. Gums become swollen and sore. Periodontal pockets have developed. Pus formation begins.
3. If no treatment is received, the inflammatory process spreads. Pockets get deeper. More pus forms. Bone loss continues.
4. Final stage. Supporting bone of the tooth has been destroyed. The tooth is lost.

Figure 3–3. **Care of teeth and gums. (From *Diabetes Forecast* 32 [4]: 1979)**

Some guidelines to alert you to the presence of periodontal disease are:

- Watch for bleeding, tender, swollen gums.
- Watch for gums that seem to pull away from the teeth.
- Be alert for loose teeth or teeth that seem to be shifting position.

To prevent periodontal disease:

- Remove plaque daily by carefully brushing and flossing your teeth.
- Visit your dentist regularly, at least every 6 months.
- Eat a well-balanced diet.
- Keep your teeth, fillings, crowns, and the like, in good repair, thus avoiding unnecessary irritation.
- Avoid clenching or grinding your teeth.
- Avoid smoking or chewing tobacco.

SKIN PROBLEMS

Individuals, whose diabetes is in good control are not more prone to skin problems than nondiabetics, but as we have seen already, diabetes is the great aggravator. Any physical problem affects diabetes, and skin problems are no exception. The key words, of course, are *good control,* and preventing problems before they occur is the best strategy.

Frequently a physician will discover diabetes because of a patient's skin problems. These may include *bacterial infections* such as styes (infections of the glands and the eyelids), boils, or carbuncles, and tenderness and inflammation around the nails. When these problems recur frequently, diabetes is usually suspected. *Localized itching* anywhere on the body, particularly in the folds of skin and in the genital area, can be caused by a yeast infection and is another common sign that alerts the physician to the possibility of diabetes.

In undetected, uncontrolled, or poorly controlled diabetes, infections develop because the skin is usually dry due to dehydration. *Dry skin* provides a fertile place for infection to develop. (Dehydration is the result of excessive urination, the body's response to the presence of high glucose in the blood.) *Poor circulation* is another factor. *Peripheral neuropathy* (nerve damage to the outer parts of the body, such as the legs and feet) which sometimes occurs in diabetes, causes some loss of sensation in this area. Because of a loss of sensation, a wound can go unnoticed until it becomes seriously infected. The body's white blood cells, which normally fight infection, seem to lose some of this ability when diabetes is uncontrolled. (This condition is reversed when diabetes is brought under good control; see chapter 8.) In uncontrolled or poorly controlled diabetes, blood glucose is high. Since infections tend to raise blood glucose also, the combination becomes a vicious cycle, one aggravating the other.

Fungus infections are thought to be more common in diabetes because of the high levels of sugar in the blood and tissues. These infections are usually found in the genital area, the armpits, on the feet, or any area aggravated by rubbing and perspiration. The principal fungi are candidiasis, also called moniliasis, a yeastlike fungus that seems to favor people with diabetes.

Diabetic dermopathy is a term describing skin problems caused by changes in the small blood vessels (microangiopathy). Other skin problems, such as bacterial and yeast infections, may indicate diabetes, but dermopathy is usually conclusive evidence of it. Diabetic dermopathy appears as light brown, scaly patches on the shins. The patches cause no pain and may be mistaken for aging spots. This skin problem is harmless and requires no treatment.

Necrobiosis lipoidica diabeticorum is somewhat like dermopathy and is also thought to be caused by blood vessel changes. While the spots usually occur on the shins they are deeper, longer, and fewer in number. They begin as a dull red raised area, slowly changing into a shiny scar with a violet border. Sometimes these spots are painful, and they can itch and crack open. This is a fairly uncommon condition and is most often found in adult women when it does occur. Occasionally the spots become ulcerated and when this happens, prompt professional attention is required to prevent infection.

Summary: The watchword for skin problems in diabetes is prevention. When any problems do occur, get professional help before an infection develops which can cause your diabetes to get out of control.

WHEN YOU ARE SICK

It happens to the healthiest of us; we get a cold, we get the flu, or other physical problems of a more serious nature arise. Any illness is a threat to diabetes control, and you should know how to deal with these problems when they arise.

The stress of illness brings about hormonal changes which may raise blood glucose and alter insulin needs. It is a mistake to think that when you use insulin or an oral drug and are ill and unable to eat, that you need not take your medication. People who take insulin or oral drugs should take their usual dose when ill. In fact, you may need to increase your insulin to compensate for the rise in blood glucose used by the illness. Those who do not take insulin may need to take it during illness to bring their diabetes under control.

Testing Is Important When You Are Ill

You may not feel like testing your blood and urine when you are ill, but it is especially important to do so at such times. For greater accuracy in testing urine, always use a second voided specimen. For people with insulin-dependent diabetes, the presence of ketones in the urine and a high blood glucose level are danger signals which mean that more insulin is needed. If untreated, this condition can lead to ketoacidosis

TABLE 3–2
FOOD FOR SICK DAYS

Easy-to-Eat Foods	Amount (for 1 Exchange)	Approximate CHO gms.	Approximate Calories
Vegetable Exchanges			
Tomato juice	½ cup	5	25
Vegetable cocktail juice	½ cup	5	25
Milk Exchanges			
Eggnog, commercial made with whole milk (nonalcoholic)	½ cup	17	170
Yogurt,* plain, made with lowfat milk	1 cup	12	120
Yogurt,* plain, made with whole milk	1 cup	12	150
Warm milk, skim	1 cup	12	90
Warm milk, lowfat	1 cup	12	120
Warm milk, whole milk	1 cup	12	150
Fruit Exchanges			
Fruit juices, unsweetened: apple, grapefruit, orange, pineapple, and apricot or peach nectar	½ cup	15	60
Grape, prune, cranberry juice cocktail	⅓ cup	15	60
Applesauce, unsweetened	½ cup	15	60
Applesauce, sweetened	¼ cup	13	50
Popsicle*	½ twin pop	12	50
Sugar,* granular	1 level tbsp.	12	45
Fat Exchanges			
Margarine	1 tsp.	0	45
Free Foods			
Fat-free broth, bouillon			
Coffee, regular or decaffeinated			
Tea			
Postum			
Starch/Bread Exchanges			
Bread, white or whole wheat, toasted or plain	1 slice	15	80
Cereal, hot	½ cup	15	80
Crackers	6 (2-in. square)	15	80
Graham crackers	3 (2½-in. square)	15	80
Ice cream (vanilla, chocolate, strawberry)	½ cup	15	170

Source: From *Diabetes Forecast* 32 (3): 1979.

*Several foods have been included under more than one list to facilitate working them into your individualized meal plan.

**When omitting bread exchange you do not need to count carbohydrate value.

TABLE 3–2 *(continued)*

Easy-to-Eat Foods	Amount (for 1 Exchange)	Approximate CHO gms.	Approximate Calories
Ice milk (vanilla, chocolate, strawberry	½ cup	15	125
Jams or jellies, regular	1 level tbsp.	14	55
Jello, regular	½ cup	18	80
Popsicle	½ twin pop	12	50
Pudding, plain (made with skim milk)	½ cup	15	80
Sherbet	¼ cup	15	80
Soft drinks, cola	6 oz.	19	75
Soft drinks, ginger ale	6 oz.	15	90
Soups, broth type	1 cup	15	80
Soups, cream type (made with water)	1 cup	15	125
Sugar, white granular	4 level tsp.	16	60
Tapioca, whole milk, plain	⅓ cup	9	75
Meat Exchanges			
Cottage cheese, any kind	¼ cup		55
Custard, baked	¼ cup (omit 1 bread exchange)**		150
Egg substitute, low cholesterol	¼ cup		50
Egg, soft-cooked or poached	1		75
Eggnog,* commercial	½ cup (omit 1 bread exchange)**		170
Yogurt,* plain, lowfat milk	1 cup (omit 1 bread exchange)**		120
Yogurt,* plain, whole milk	1 cup (omit 1 bread exchange)**		150

and coma. Ketoacidosis occurs when there is not enough insulin, and the body uses its stores of fat in place of glucose, causing ketones to appear in the urine (see chapter 6). When blood and urine tests show a combination of high glucose and ketones, call your doctor promptly.

People with non-insulin-dependent diabetes do not usually show ketones in the urine. If you aren't feeling well and your blood or urine tests have been high in glucose for 24 hours, you should be in touch with your doctor. It is possible for Type II patients to develop hyperosmolar coma (a coma caused by dehydration and loss of fluid; see chapter 6). Vomiting, nausea, and diarrhea are always causes for concern since they can result in extreme loss of fluid. Report these symptoms to your doctor promptly.

Below are some tips to help you when you are sick:

1. Take your usual dose of insulin or oral drug, and test your blood or urine.
2. If your tests are high in glucose and show ketones, call your doctor.
3. If you use insulin, be sure to have a reserve supply of Regular insulin on hand should your doctor prescribe it.
4. Follow your meal plan as closely as possible. Eating and drinking are important. If you have difficulty eating, try the soft or liquid foods shown in table 3–2.
5. Vomiting, nausea, and diarrhea are danger signals and should be reported to your doctor immediately.
6. Know how to take your temperature.
7. If you live alone, notify a friend or relative that you are ill.
8. When you are sick for more than one day, call your doctor for advice on what to do. Discuss the use of any nonprescription drugs you are using.

4

LIFETIME CONSIDERATIONS

ALCOHOL

To drink or not to drink is a dilemma often faced by people with diabetes. The drinking of alcoholic beverages is a well-established social custom. As social creatures we are bound to encounter many occasions when alcohol is served. There is no evidence that a single drink shortly before dinner or a glass of wine with dinner will harm a diabetic in good control. If you choose to drink, discuss with your doctor or diet counselor how alcohol can be fitted into your meal plan. Although alcohol is made from carbohydrates, it is digested like a fat in the body and is classified as a Fat Exchange when calculated in the diabetic diet (see table 4–1).

How Alcohol Affects the Body

Alcohol is a drug that can be toxic to the body. When used to excess it dehydrates the body, irritates the mucous membranes, causes nerve damage, and adversely affects the digestive, central nervous, and cardiovascular systems; it raises blood cholesterol and it lowers blood sugar. When ingested it goes directly from the digestive tract to the liver, where it is metabolized (changed into energy). When the liver is processing alcohol it is unable to release its own stores of glycogen, the body's reserve supply of sugar. This can spell trouble for the insulin-dependent person by hastening a hypoglycemic/insulin reaction.

Alcohol can affect persons who take oral drugs too, causing dizziness, flushing, and nausea. Alcohol has no nutritional value but does have calories that must be calculated in the diet. It tends to affect judgment, making it easier to overdo on snacks when drinking. For anyone following a calorie-restricted diet this can be disastrous.

Whether you choose to drink or not is for you and your doctor to decide, but if you do drink you should know the rules.

1. Always eat something when you drink. Alcohol lowers blood glucose, and eating will help avoid hypoglycemic reactions. The main cause of hypoglycemia when drinking is an omitted or delayed meal.
2. Limit the number of your drinks to one or two.
3. Avoid sweet wines, liqueurs, and sweetened mixes.
4. Drink slowly.
5. When you drink, don't drive. A hypoglycemic reaction might be mistaken for drunkenness, and proper treatment could be delayed.

TABLE 4–1
ALCOHOL, CALORIES, AND EXCHANGES

	Serving Size	Approximate Calories	Number of Exchanges
Distilled Spirits (86 Proof)	1½ oz.	107	2½ fats
Dry Table Wine (12% alcohol)	3 oz.	68	1½ fats
Regular Beer (4.5% alcohol)	12 oz.	151	3½ fats or 2 fats + 1 bread
"Light" Beer (3.5% alcohol)	12 oz.	97	2 fats

Source: From *Diabetes Forecast* 33 (6): 1980.

When You Don't Drink

Many persons with diabetes decide not to drink. What are your alternatives? Today there are a variety of "waters" such as mineral, spring, or sparkling, natural water, or your favorite diet soda. If you don't drink, don't apologize. Whether you are watching your weight or your diabetes, you can very gracefully ask for a nonalcoholic beverage without embarrassment today. Nonalcoholic drinks are available in any bar or restaurant, and a thoughtful hostess will serve them too.

SMOKING

In 1964 the U.S. Surgeon General warned Americans of the dangers of cigarette smoking. The public education program launched by that announcement has been so widespread that there can be no doubt in anyone's mind at this time that smoking is a hazard to health.

Smoking predisposes the body to chronic bronchitis, emphysema, and lung cancer. The chemicals in cigarette smoke narrow the blood vessels, and since people with diabetes are prone to cardiovascular disease anyway, smoking is particularly dangerous for them. To avoid smoking if you have diabetes just makes good sense. If you don't smoke, don't start. It is said that an addiction to cigarette smoking is more difficult to break than an addiction to heroin.

If you smoke, stop. There are self-help groups in almost every community. Consult the yellow pages of your local telephone directory for the group nearest you. Joining one of these groups will help to rid you of a dangerous habit which is costly not only in dollars, but more important, to your health.

Young people frequently ask if smoking marijuana will aggravate their diabetes. All of the statements about cigarette smoking apply equally to smoking marijuana. Studies have shown that marijuana tends to alter judgment, weakens the body's reserves against infections, and promotes the "munchies," uncontrolled snacking. People with diabetes need to pay particular attention to good health habits, and smoking pot or cigarettes will not only jeopardize your general health but your diabetes too.

DRIVING

People who *qualify* can drive a car. How do you qualify if you have diabetes? Just like anyone else, you apply for a driver's license. For young people applying for their first license, a driver's education class, usually given in high school, will provide the necessary mechanical knowledge for handling a car and teach the rules of the road. When applying for a license, be truthful and say you have diabetes. All 50 states permit people with diabetes to drive. Some states may require a medical statement saying that your diabetes is in good control and there are no serious complications that would interfere with driving.

Are There Any Driving Restrictions?

Yes. Insulin-dependent people currently cannot be licensed to drive commercial vehicles (trucks, buses, etc.) engaged in interstate or foreign commerce. This is a federal regulation (see section on Careers on the next page).

As in all other aspects of living with diabetes, but particularly when driving, it is necessary to avoid hypoglycemia. Always keep some form of sugar handy. Never skip a meal. A good rule for the road, when driving all day, is to stop and eat 10 grams of carbohydrate every hour, such as an orange, two graham crackers, or six lifesavers. If you feel the symptoms of an insulin reaction coming, pull off the road immediately and eat some sugar. Follow this with a snack of crackers and cheese, or a sandwich to keep the blood sugar level up.

Always wear identification, and keep a sticker on the dashboard of your car which says, "I have diabetes." You should also carry an identification card in your wallet which says you have diabetes, as an added precaution.

People with uncontrolled diabetes should never drive. If your control has been poor, move over and let someone else take the wheel. Fluctuating blood sugar can affect vision and judgment. In case of an accident, don't use diabetes or hypoglycemia as an excuse if that was not the case. Doing so will only make it harder on others should they ever find themselves in a similar situation.

In Summary:

- Learn to be a good driver by proper education and strict attention to the rules of the road.
- Avoid an insulin reaction by eating a snack at regular intervals when driving.
- Never skip a meal in an attempt to get to your destination more quickly.
- Pull off the road and stop immediately if you feel the symptoms of an insulin reaction.
- Wear identification and keep a sticker prominently displayed in your car saying that you have diabetes.

CAREERS AND EMPLOYMENT

When you are young and choosing a career, deciding what you will do with your life is probably one of the most important decisions you will ever make. There are many careers open to you, but some are better suited to you individually than others. People with diabetes work productively in a wide variety of professions, trades, and other occupations. If you are in high school discuss your preferences with your parents, your guidance counselor, and your physician. These are the people who know your particular strengths and weaknesses.

There are a few types of work that may not be best for you. For example, being a policeman, fireman, airline ground or flight attendant may not be wise career choices because such jobs are likely to have erratic hours. Any job with fairly regular hours is more desirable than one with a swing shift that changes every week or two.

The American Diabetes Association believes that any person with diabetes who is seeking employment should be given consideration based solely upon his or her individual qualifications to perform the specific duties involved. Certain changes in federal and state laws require that employers give equal job opportunities to qualified "handicapped" persons. These laws include people who have diabetes. Check with your local ADA Affiliate for details about the laws that apply to your state and the job you are considering.

A few jobs are currently not open to you. Under present Armed Service regulations, insulin-dependent diabetes disqualifies a person from entering any branch of the armed forces. The Civil Air regulations of the Federal Aviation Administration state that diabetes requiring insulin for control disqualifies a person from getting a pilot's license. Department of Transportation regulations prohibit insulin-dependent people from driving vehicles in interstate or foreign commerce. Each of these policies is under review.

Make Your First Job Count

Your first job may be one you take before completing your formal education; a summer, after-school, or evening job. Any work that does not interfere with your diabetes control is suitable, although you may need to adjust your daily schedule to accommodate your job. To be comfortable on the job, it is best to tell your employer and those you work with that you have diabetes and what they can do if an insulin reaction should occur. Show them the sugar that you carry. You may think this is a risk to your job, but if you do maintain good control of your diabetes and perform the job in a superior manner, you will be proof positive that people with diabetes are desirable workers. Be regular in attendance, report to work on time, and never use your diabetes as an excuse for poor performance.

Starting Out in Your Chosen Career

When you have finished your education and are looking for a career opportunity, explore the kinds of jobs for which you are qualified and those in which you are most likely to succeed. If you have planned your education wisely, and prepared well for your chosen career, then diabetes should present no problems. But you still have to land that first job.

The following are some things to remember as you enter the work force for the first time.

1. Maintain your diabetes in good control. If your employer asks for a physical examination, you will have no problem showing that your diabetes won't interfere with your performance of the job.
2. Be honest with your future employer. If you are straightforward in volunteering the information that you have diabetes, he or she will admire you for it. Not mentioning the fact could be embarrassing at some future time and could be grounds for dismissal.
3. Be informed and prepared to discuss diabetes and how it will affect your work. A good record of part-time employment will help.
4. Be positive. Don't regard your diabetes as a defect, and don't ask for special consideration because of it.
5. Apply for jobs for which you are qualified.
6. When you are hired, be the best. Learn all you can about the job; be punctual, don't miss work unless absolutely necessary. If you have the flu, for example, and are absent from work, tell your employer why you were absent so he will know it wasn't your diabetes that kept you at home.

Changing Careers

A number of years ago John Murphy, a commercial pilot, was discovered to have diabetes that required insulin for control.

Flying was the only thing he knew. He had been an Air Force pilot in World War II. He loved flying, and so it was natural for him to become a commercial pilot when peace came. The diagnosis of diabetes was devastating when it came, but his doctor very bluntly told him, "It's your job or your life." John started selling mutual funds. He later confessed that learning a new career in midlife wasn't half as hard as giving up flying. He ultimately became a top salesman for his company. He feels that the self-discipline required to live with diabetes helped him to put his life in perspective and that he has lived a healthier life because of it.

If your diabetes necessitates a change in your career, and you are unable to afford the expense of college courses or retraining, training in a new skill is available to persons with diabetes through State Departments of Vocational Rehabilitation. Your local American Diabetes Association Affiliate will help you find the programs that are available in your state.

Discrimination in Employment

Unfortunately, discrimination against diabetic people does exist, although it is much less common today than it was even a few years ago. Title V of the Rehabilitation Act of 1973 states that you cannot be turned down for a job for which you are qualified just because you have diabetes. The law applies to all departments and agencies of the federal government, the U.S. postal system, and the Service Rate Commission. It also applies to contractors or subcontractors who receive $2,500 or more in federal money per year. This includes many businesses and industries throughout the country.

The following are actions you can take under the law if you have been denied a promotion or rejected for employment because you have diabetes.

1. First, discuss the issues with your employer or the employment manager who rejected your application.
2. If this proves unsuccessful, you can file a written complaint to the Handicapped Workers Task Force,

Department of Labor, 200 Constitution Avenue, N.E., Washington, D.C. 20210. You will be notified of their findings and any agreement they reach with your employer.

3. If the Department of Labor rejects your complaint, you can ask for a review.

4. If the Department of Labor agrees that your complaint is valid, they will ask your employer to state in writing that he will take corrective action. The employer may ask for and be given a hearing. If the hearing is not favorable to him, he can lose his existing and future government contracts or be fined.

INSURANCE

How to Get Insurance When You Have Diabetes

With the rising costs of medical care today, it is important that every family have health insurance. This is especially true if you have diabetes. Even in the well-controlled person, treatment in a hospital may sometimes be required. It is possible for you to get health insurance through group plans. Most employers provide such plans, and spouses and children under 19 years of age are usually covered by these plans.

Group plans are almost always offered for a definite enrollment period. It is best to apply as soon as you know that a plan is open. Although persons with diabetes are admitted, there may be a waiting period before expenses pertaining to diabetes are covered. Be sure to read your policy for "preexisting" conditions (any illness that was present before you purchased the policy).

A basic group health plan will usually cover medical expenses for in-hospital treatment, doctor's charges, and drugs. Plans do vary however; some pay 100 percent, while others require the policy holder to pay 20 to 25 percent of the total cost. The plan may have a straight deductible (the

portion you pay before the insurance company takes over)
wherein the patient pays for the first $50 or $100 of the cost,
and the insurance company pays the remainder. Some basic
plans cover outpatient costs and doctor's office visits. The
best way to find out what your policy includes is to read it
carefully, then go over it with your employer or the agent who
is offering the plan.

Major medical group insurance plans are available to
diabetic people, their children, and spouses if applied for
during the open enrollment period. This kind of insurance is
difficult and costly to obtain on an individual basis. Major
medical plans usually cover most medical charges, doctor's
office visits, prescribed medicines, insulin, syringes, and oral
drugs. If the plan has a deductible, these expenses are paid
by the insurance company after the patient has paid his
portion. Strips for self-monitoring of blood glucose are generally covered, and in some cases, the meters are also covered.

Diabetes education is a vital element in the control of
diabetes, and some plans will pay for it when it is offered in
the hospital, in the doctor's office, or in the outpatient clinic,
while some plans cover only in-hospital education.

What about Life Insurance?

There are two basic types of life insurance, and depending
upon your age and responsibilities, you may want to look into
both types. One is *term insurance* which is bought for a
specified number of years, usually 1, 5, 10, or 20 years or up
to age 65 or 70. At the end of the specified time the insurance
company has the right to refuse to renew the policy.

Whole life insurance costs more than term insurance, but
it covers you until death, and it cannot be terminated by the
insurance company unless you neglect to pay the premiums.
You can always obtain a loan on this type of policy, and the
loan can be of indefinite duration when necessary. Any un-
paid loan balance is deducted from the face value when the
policy is paid out.

Things to remember when you are seeking life insurance: shop around, talk to several insurance agents, and read the policy very carefully before signing. The American Diabetes Association suggests that you submit a "trial application" first. This means that the insurance company will review your application and then inform you whether or not they will accept you. If you are turned down on a trial application, this will not harm your chances for acceptance by some other insurance company. Submit a formal application only after you find a company that wants you and a policy that you feel gives you the best coverage. You must state on the application that you have diabetes. Not to do so might cause your policy to be invalid. You can get insurance, but you need to know where to look for it.

TRAVEL

As one young person said rather wistfully, "I'm going on vacation, and just for once I'd like to leave my diabetes behind." This echoes the feelings of many people with diabetes. However, with a little careful planning you can jet off to Tahiti, backpack in the Sierras, or bicycle around Europe; whatever your heart desires and your pocketbook allows can be yours—*with* diabetes (fig. 4–1).

Before You Start

1. Have a medical examination to be sure your diabetes is in good control.
2. Get a letter from your doctor saying that you have diabetes. You may not need it, but it will save time and questions, particularly if you are carrying syringes with you.
3. Get prescriptions from your doctor for insulin, syringes, oral drugs if you take them (prescription regulations vary from state to state in the United States),

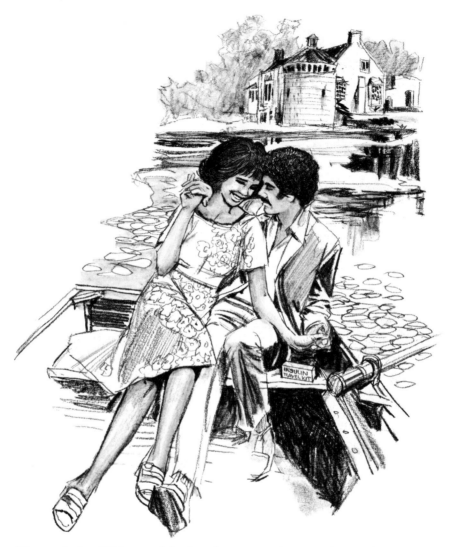

Figure 4–1. **With careful planning, one can travel anywhere, any-time—even with diabetes.**

antidiarrheal medicines, and any other medicines that you may need.

4. If your travel plans extend beyond two weeks have a dental checkup if you haven't seen your dentist lately. What is worse than a toothache in a strange city or on top of a high mountain?

5. If you are traveling in the United States call your local American Diabetes Affiliate and get a list of affiliates in the areas where you will be visiting. This will be useful in case of emergency. If you are traveling abroad ask for a list of the International Diabetes Federation organizations. There are offices in most foreign countries, and should you need medical attention these organizations could be helpful. You can usually get the name of an English-speaking physician from the American Embassy or Consulate of your host country.

6. Get all necessary immunizations at least one month prior to departure. If you should have a reaction that disturbs your diabetes control, this will give you time to stabilize it before leaving.

Pack Your Bags

If you are traveling by bus, car, train, or plane pack the following items in a carryall bag which you *keep with you* at all times.

1. All the insulin you will need for the trip. (U-100 insulin is sold only in the United States, Canada, Australia, and New Zealand.) Insulin is very stable and does not need to be refrigerated. It should be protected from extremes of temperature above 90 and below 35 degrees. A good rule to remember is that any temperature your body can stand comfortably, your insulin can also stand. Never pack your insulin in a bag that will be stowed in the luggage compartment of an airplane because it could freeze or be lost.

2. Take all the syringes you will need with you. Disposable syringes are best for travel. This is necessary because buying syringes with an out-of-state prescription can be difficult. Abroad, U-100 syringes are only sold in those countries where the insulin is available, namely Canada, Australia, and New Zealand.

3. Take your blood and urine testing materials with you.

4. If you take oral drugs, take your entire supply with you. If you are traveling abroad it might be a good idea to take a little extra in case you are delayed in returning home. Products differ, and you could risk your diabetes control by switching to a new product.

5. Take all other drugs and medical supplies that you may need, including ready glucose, glucagon, antidiarrheal medicines, alcohol, and cotton swabs. You don't want to waste precious vacation time looking for a drug store in a strange city.

6. Always wear and carry identification saying that you have diabetes. This is true whether you go to the corner grocery store or to the far corners of the earth. You should have a card for your purse or wallet showing you are diabetic and what medication you take. You should also have some type of wearable identification such as a bracelet or necklace in case your purse or wallet is stolen.

7. Carry a well-wrapped, airtight snack pack containing some carbohydrate and some protein—crackers, cheese, peanut butter, fruit, and some form of sugar— in case of an insulin reaction. This can be replenished as needed and will be invaluable when a meal is delayed.

8. Take clothes appropriate for the vacation; at least one pair of comfortable shoes, sun glasses, and sun tan lotion.

Tips for Insulin Users

If you are taking a long trip across time zones, discuss with your doctor before you leave how to schedule your injections and meals. If your flight requires an in-flight injection at high altitudes, put less air in the insulin bottle than usual, perhaps only half as much as the number of units you intend to draw. At high altitudes, there is greater pressure in the insulin bottle, even though the cabin is pressurized. When traveling by plane you can order your meals in advance, requesting the hour at which you need to be served. If the service is delayed for any reason, you can always resort to your carefully stocked snack pack stowed away in your hand luggage.

Travel by ship, car, bus, or train will present no time change problems, since the variations in time will never be more than one or two hours per day. When traveling by any of these modes of transportation however, it is important that you keep to your regular mealtime schedule. When traveling by car, if you are the driver you should eat approximately 10 grams of carbohydrate every hour. This could be an orange, or two graham crackers, or six lifesavers.

No matter how you travel, you should exercise regularly. If you are traveling on an airplane or a train get up frequently and walk up and down the aisles. When traveling by bus, stops are usually made every two hours. You should take advantage of these stops to get out and stretch your legs and walk around. When traveling by automobile, you can stop to eat your snack and exercise wherever you want to, but every two hours is recommended. Travel by ship provides every opportunity for a variety of exercise.

Write It All Down

No matter how well you plan, your diabetes schedule may be interrupted. At the start of the trip it is a good idea to keep a careful record of the times of your injections, meals, your urine test results, or your blood glucose readings if you monitor your blood. If you see a pattern of either high or low blood sugar, you can make adjustments to your schedule. Keeping your diabetes under good control will make your vacation more enjoyable.

Once you have arrived at your destination, remember to adjust your insulin dose and food intake to the type of physical activity your plans involve. Sitting on a sightseeing bus is different from skiing, hiking, or swimming. Eating something like fruit, crackers, milk, or ice cream before commencing a strenuous activity will help to ward off an insulin reaction.

Eating and Drinking Away from Home

You have already learned the basics of eating away from home. When you travel, especially to foreign countries, trying exotic foods is part of the fun. As long as you know your prescribed meal plan and how to make substitutions, you should have no trouble. In South and Central America and Asia do not eat raw meats or fish, milk or milk products, unpeeled fruits, lettuce or other raw vegetables, water, or ice cubes. Bottled drinking water is usually available but if not, tea and coffee are generally safe because the water has been boiled.

Even the best plans sometimes go wrong. Emergencies can happen. Tell your traveling companions you have diabetes. Describe to them how you act when having an insulin reaction. Show them the sugar, ready glucose, and glucagon you carry and how these are used. If you become ill while traveling, check your urine for glucose and ketones four times a day or monitor your blood. Follow the instructions given you by your physician. If illness is prolonged for more than a day, contact a doctor or go to a hospital for treatment.

Summary: When you travel with diabetes, be prepared. Your trip will be more enjoyable if your diabetes is kept under good control. Follow your physician's instructions on how to adjust your insulin and meals to meet time changes and extra physical activity. Stick as closely as possible to your regular meal plan and meal time schedule. Always carry and wear identification. Alert your traveling companions to the fact that you have diabetes and how they can help you. In case of an emergency, contact a doctor or go to the hospital for treatment.

Bon voyage and happy landings!

MARRIAGE AND PREGNANCY

Many young people wonder, "Should I marry? How will diabetes affect my marriage? Will I pass diabetes on to my children?" These are wise and thoughtful questions. When contemplating marriage the young person with diabetes should discuss frankly with his/her future spouse the responsibilities and self-discipline that diabetes entails. In addition to the physical and emotional aspects of diabetes, the economic factors need to be considered. A willingness on the part of the nondiabetic partner to learn as much as possible about diabetes and to accept the fact that there will be added responsibilities and extra expense because of diabetes, will help prepare the way for any rough spots ahead. No marriage is without problems, but a burden shared is a burden halved. When both partners start out with a full knowledge and mature understanding of diabetes and the responsibilities involved, fewer problems will arise.

Should We Have Children?

"What are the chances that our children will become diabetic?" The most recent research indicates that if only one parent has Type I diabetes the chance that the children will develop Type I diabetes is less than 10 percent. When both parents have diabetes the possibility is less than 50 percent. If there is diabetes on both sides of the family, but neither parent has diabetes, development of diabetes by the children is less predictable. The inheritance of diabetes is now thought to be "multifactorial," meaning a combination or coming together of many different inherited factors. The prevalence of Type II diabetes in families tends to be higher than Type I diabetes. It is important to remember, when Type II diabetes is evident in your family background, that this type of diabetes can probably be avoided, or the onset delayed, by maintaining ideal body weight throughout your lifetime.

When deciding whether or not to have a family, a young couple might like to keep in mind that the child inherits not one but many traits from both parents, of which diabetes might be just one. Should the possibility of passing a single trait deny the world of such artists as Mario Lanza or Paul Cezanne, or geniuses such as Thomas Edison?

Along these same lines it is now estimated that one in four persons carries the diabetic trait, although they may not know it. A carrier may pass the trait on to his or her children but will probably not develop diabetes. If this theory is correct, and even if no children were born to known diabetic people in the future, the number of diabetic people in the world would not be significantly changed.

Some people with diabetes prefer to adopt children. While the number of adoptable babies has declined somewhat, adoption is still possible. Raising a family is an extra challenge to your diabetes. Being a parent makes physical and emotional demands upon you, but it has rewards too. Once you have made your decision, however, you have crossed the psychological barrier and are on your way to success. The more carefully a couple considers their options, the wiser their decision will be.

Pregnancy

If you decide to have a baby, plan ahead. The prospective mother should have her diabetes under good control several months before becoming pregnant. Closely monitored diabetic pregnancies today are 95 percent successful, compared with 98 to 99 percent for nondiabetics. Your baby will have the best chance if you keep your blood glucose as close to normal as possible all during your pregnancy.

Before you become pregnant discuss your plans with your physician. If possible, put yourself in the hands of a team of experts consisting of a diabetologist, obstetrician, nurse clinician, and dietitian. This type of help is available at many larger hospitals, and the closer you are physically, emotionally, and personally to your team, the easier it will be for you. The care of a diabetic pregnancy is expensive; therefore, careful planning, along with a good health and major medical insurance plan, will make it easier. You and your husband should examine your health insurance policy and make sure exactly when your maternity benefits begin. Some policies have clauses that do not provide coverage until after the policy has been in force for a year. Knowing the cost before your baby is conceived will give you both more peace of mind, and this will be reflected in your diabetes control.

Each trimester (3-month period) of pregnancy is important. The first three months are critical to fetal development, since this is when the formation of your baby's organs takes place. This is also the time when abnormalities are most likely to occur, so it is imperative that your control be optimal those first few weeks even before you know for certain that you are pregnant.

Your control, for the most part, will be up to you. Your doctor will decide the best method for you. This may involve urine tests or blood tests taken at home, and you may be given an insulin infusion pump to help you stay in better control. These latter methods are very new, require strict attention and discipline on your part, but do pay off in having a healthy baby, because of almost minute-to-minute control of blood glucose. (The insulin pump is worn around the waist and provides a constant infusion of small amounts of insulin, with a self-adjusting device for larger doses at mealtimes.)

During the last half of pregnancy your baby grows dramatically, and your need for insulin will probably increase. In the nondiabetic mother this is the time in pregnancy when gestational diabetes may appear. When this happens the doctor or dietitian will provide you with guidelines for keeping your blood glucose under control. In some cases, gestational diabetes is treated with insulin. An evaluation after pregnancy will be made. A person who has gestational diabetes is at risk for developing diabetes later in life and should have periodic checkups thereafter.

During the third trimester diabetes control and physician follow-up are crucial. Your doctor may require an "estriol" test. Estriol is a hormone produced by the fetus (developing baby) and the placenta (membranes attached to the lining of the uterus). Estriol is measured by testing either the blood or urine of the mother. If the level of estriol is normal, your baby is most likely healthy. The baby's heartbeat will also be monitored, and this is the time when some women are given an amniocentesis test in which a tiny amount of amniotic fluid (fluid that surrounds the fetus) is withdrawn. This test shows, among other things, the maturity of the baby's lungs and whether or not the baby will be able to breathe normally after delivery. An ultrasound test, which detects sounds and movements inside the body, may be performed one or more times during pregnancy to determine the baby's growth. The ultrasonic technique used is similar to that employed in tracking a submarine.

Expectant mothers with diabetes are often hospitalized for a variable time before the expected delivery date and may be required to stay longer than nondiabetic mothers. If complications occur, hospitalization before delivery may be longer. These precautions are taken to insure a safe delivery and a healthy mother and child.

Summary: When you marry, both of you should have a full knowledge of diabetes and an understanding of the added responsibilities that diabetes entails: physical, emotional, and financial. The nondiabetic partner should be willing to share these responsibilities and make any sacrifices that the self-discipline of diabetes requires. If you decide to have children, plan ahead. A woman should have her diabetes under good control long before pregnancy occurs.

5

TYPE I, INSULIN-DEPENDENT DIABETES

The goals in the treatment of insulin-dependent diabetes are to provide sufficient nutrition/food for growth and development of the body; to attain and maintain ideal body weight; to keep blood glucose levels as near to normal as possible; and to prevent the complications of diabetes insofar as present knowledge permits. This is accomplished by a balance of food, exercise, and insulin.

Always keep in mind that eating and digesting food raise the blood glucose level; activity and insulin lower it. Once you have injected insulin, it is inside your body lowering your blood glucose at a given rate of speed, for eight hours or longer. Like a nonstop train it travels through your bloodstream. You need to eat at regular intervals to keep the train moving at a safe speed. If you take your insulin and forget to eat, your blood glucose will fall below normal, and you will have an insulin reaction. If you eat, but neglect to take your insulin, your blood glucose will rise above normal.

While keeping a regular schedule of meals, injections, and exercise may be difficult to get used to at first, you will soon be able to fit it into your daily activities. If your mind forgets, your body will remind you with signals of low or high blood sugar (see chapter 6.) And, as has already been stressed, avoiding the "swings" of blood glucose to either higher or lower than normal is what good control in diabetes is all about.

Your meal plan will be designed to include carbohydrates, proteins, and fats, distributed throughout the day to provide available glucose when your insulin is most active. Figure 5–1 shows the differences in 24-hour blood glucose response to injections of short-, intermediate-, and long-acting insulins.

Your physician or diet counselor will work out a meal plan for you to suit your needs, taking into consideration your age, your occupation, your daily activity, medication, and exercise. The plan will probably call for three meals and two or three snacks at certain hours of the day. This plan may need to be changed from time to time to allow for growth, change in activities, and other factors. As you learn to follow your

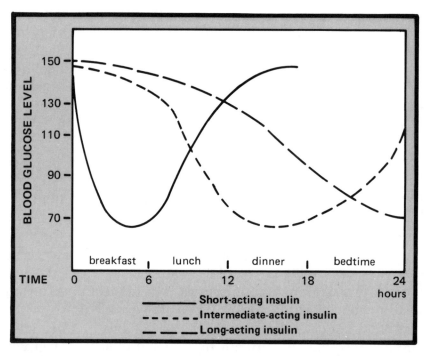

Figure 5–1. **Blood glucose response to the injection of three types of insulin.**

meal plan you can observe how well it works for you. If you have periods of hunger, or experience symptoms of an insulin reaction at particular times of the day, these should be reported to your doctor so that an adjustment can be made.

INSULIN

Insulin is one of many hormones produced in the pancreas of humans and other animals. Its primary job is to regulate blood-glucose levels. But people with Type I diabetes do not produce their own insulin; they rely on insulin from other sources, primarily pigs and cows, and increasingly, from genetics laboratories. This insulin is injected into the fatty tissue of the skin and is subsequently absorbed into the bloodstream.

When Drs. Banting and Best discovered insulin in 1921, they found Regular or short-acting insulin. Since then, other substances have been added to alter insulin's action. Today there are several types of insulin available. Your doctor will choose the one that is best for you, but you should be familiar with the different types of insulins and how they act.

Key words you will need to understand are action time, onset, peak, and duration. *Action time* refers to how quickly insulin reaches the bloodstream and affects the blood-glucose level. *Onset* refers to the time it begins to affect the blood-glucose level (1 hour after the injection or 12 hours). *Peak* refers to the time during which the insulin is most effective at lowering the blood glucose level. (In most cases, you'll want insulin to be peaking during or just after a meal.) *Duration* refers to the length of time that insulin remains in the bloodstream. While these terms may sound similar, their individual importance becomes clear when you consider the cumulative effects of taking insulin for long periods of time or using multiple injections.

Types of Insulins

There are three types of insulins: Regular or short-acting, intermediate-acting, and long-acting. Table 5–1 provides the names of insulins currently available in the United States. (It is important to remember that individuals will have a unique reaction to insulin, so times are only approximate.)

Regular or short-acting insulin usually reaches the bloodstream within 30 minutes. Its peak can be anywhere from 1 to 5 hours after injection. This type of insulin remains in the bloodstream for about 8 to 16 hours. This insulin is usually called Regular with a capital R. Short-acting insulins are clear.

A special type of Regular insulin is called Semilente. It usually takes one to two hours to affect blood glucose, peaks 3 to 8 hours after injection, and lasts 10 to 16 hours.

Intermediate-acting insulin usually reaches the bloodstream about 90 minutes after the injection. It peaks 4 to 12 hours after injection, and stays in the blood for about 24 hours. Intermediate-acting (and long-acting) insulins are suspensions. (Suspensions are fluids with particles mixed in, but not dissolved.) Extra ingredients have been added to slow the release of insulin into the body and prolong its action. Insulin suspensions are cloudy, which means all intermediate- and long-acting insulins are cloudy.

There are two varieties of intermediate-acting insulins: Lente and NPH. Lente insulin's action is prolonged by zinc. It is either called Lente or L insulin. NPH insulin is prolonged by zinc and protamine, a fish protein. It is called NPH or N.

Long-acting insulins take 4 to 6 hours to reach the bloodstream, are strongest 14 to 24 hours after injection, and stay in the blood for up to 36 hours. Most experts believe that long-acting insulins do not peak in the blood the same way the short or intermediate-acting insulins do. However, combined with other insulins, they are quite effective at lowering blood-glucose levels and can contribute to hypoglycemic episodes.

There are two types of long-acting insulin: Ultralente, sometimes just called U, and PZI. Ultralente's prolonged action is due to additional zinc, while PZI's is due to zinc and protamine.

Source, Purity, Cost

Today, three types of insulin are available: pork, beef, or human, which comes in two forms—semisynthetic (made by converting pork insulin to a form identical to human insulin), and "recombinant" or rDNA (a form identical to human insulin made through genetic engineering). The human-type insulins have just come onto the market during the 1980s but are expected to become more popular.

The source for the insulin has little to do with how well it works on lowering blood glucose. However, the source can affect how quickly the body absorbs the insulin. The newer "human" insulins (semisynthetic and recombinant) appear to be absorbed faster than the beef or pork mixtures.

Purity can also affect how well insulin is absorbed. Highly purified pork insulins and particularly the human insulins appear to cause fewer allergic reactions and other side effects.

Insulin has been an expensive drug and will continue to be for a while. That's because it had to be extracted from the pancreases of slaughtered cattle and hogs. It takes about 10,000 pounds of raw pancreases to produce one pound of pure zinc insulin crystals, which then have to be purified further. This means that it takes a lot of raw material to produce a little of the final product and, consequently, the whole process is very expensive. However, the introduction of genetic engineering into this marketplace is expected to lower the price.

As stated earlier, your doctor will select the insulin that will best suit your needs. You should never switch insulins without your doctor's guidance, as onset and action times can vary and your entire diabetes regimen must be adjusted

TABLE 5-1 _____
INSULIN ACTION

Rapid-Acting (onset 1/2–4 hours, duration 5–16 hours)

Humulin Regular
Novolin R (Regular)
    (formerly Actrapid Human)
Velosulin (Regular)
Iletin II Regular
Iletin II Regular
Purified Pork R (Regular)
    (formerly Actrapid)
Velosulin (Regular)
Purified Pork S (Semilente)
    (formerly Semitard)
Iletin I Regular
Regular
Iletin I Semilente
Semilente

Intermediate-Acting (onset 1–4 hours, duration 16–28 hours)

Humulin L
Humulin NPH
Insulatard+ (NPH)
Novolin L (Lente)
    (formerly Monotard Human)
Novolin N (NPH)
Iletin II Lente
Iletin II NPH
Iletin II Lente
Iletin II NPH
Insulatard (NPH)
Purified Pork Lente
    (formerly Monotard)
Purified Pork N (NPH)
    (formerly Protaphane)
Iletin I Lente
Iletin I NPH
NPH

Long-Acting (onset 4–6 hours, duration 36 hours)

Iletin II PZI
Iletin II PZI
Purified Beef U (Ultralente)
    (formerly Ultratard)
Iletin I PZI

Source: From *Diabetes Forecast* 39 (3): 1986.

TABLE 5–1 *(continued)*

Iletin I Ultralente
Ultralente

Mixtures

Mixtard + 30%
(30% Regular, 70% NPH)

accordingly. If cost is a consideration, discuss this with your doctor as well.

Syringes

The advent of disposable plastic syringes has saved many people's time and energy. Years ago, glass syringes had to be sterilized after every use and meticulously cared for in between. Today's lightweight, plastic disposables can be tossed after the microfine needle is broken.

Many people reuse these disposable syringes without any problem. If you reuse a disposable, recap the needle immediately after use. The syringe and needle can be stored in the refrigerator, but this is not necessary. Many experts recommend using the syringe only twice, as the needle will become dull.

Insulin Pumps

You may have heard or read about the insulin pump, a small (pocket-calculator size) computerized device that delivers insulin in a slow, steady dose throughout the day, and allows the user to program for extra insulin at mealtimes. The pump, often worn on a belt around the waist, works like this: Insulin flows from the storage vial in the pump through a plastic tube and into a needle that is placed in the abdomen, flank, or thigh. The needle remains in place 1 to 3 days. To accommodate bathing, swimming, or strenuous exercise, the wearer can remove the pump and cap the needle.

The pump has been very helpful in improving control for individuals who are highly motivated to maintain tight control of diabetes. However, the pump is not for everyone. If you are interested in this type of therapy, discuss it with your doctor.

Be Advised: The American Diabetes Association recommends that individuals who use insulin pumps be under the care of a physician who is familiar with insulin-pump therapy.

INSULIN INJECTION TECHNIQUES

In order to offset the effect of food on the blood glucose level, insulin should be taken about 30 minutes before a meal. The following illustrations show step-by-step procedures for insulin injection.

1. Wash your hands with soap and water. Assemble all the things you will need for your injection; that is, alcohol, cotton swabs, syringe, and insulin.

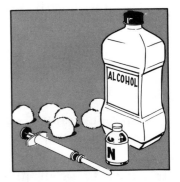

Figure 5–2.1

2. Wipe off the top of the insulin bottle with a cotton swab dipped in alcohol.

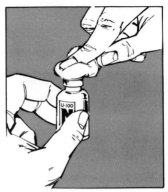

Figure 5–2.2

3. If you use a glass syringe, assemble it, making certain that you do not touch the plunger or the needle. If you use a disposable syringe, unwrap it and remove the needle guard without touching the needle.

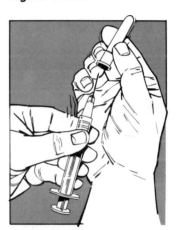

Figure 5–2.3

4. Pull the plunger back (draw air into the syringe) to the unit mark corresponding to the number of units in your dose.

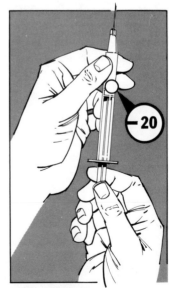

Figure 5–2.4

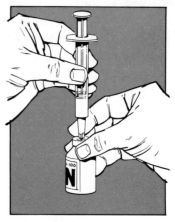

5. With the bottle right-side up, push the needle into the center of the rubber cap on the insulin bottle.

Figure 5–2.5

6. Push the plunger down so that all the air in the syringe is transferred to the air space inside of the bottle.

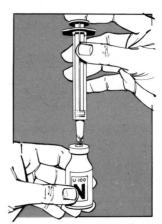

Figure 5–2.6

7. Turn the bottle upside-down with the needle still in it; slowly pull the plunger back to 2 or 3 units more than your dose and allow the insulin to flow into the syringe.

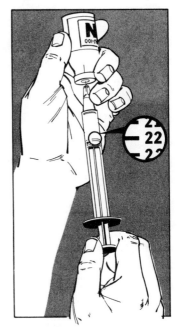

Figure 5–2.7

8. Flick your finger against the syringe lightly to remove any air bubbles.

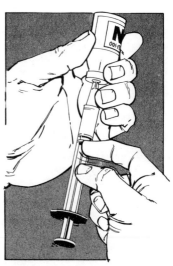

Figure 5–2.8

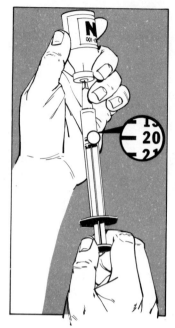

9. Push the plunger to your exact dose. Air injected into the body is not harmful, but it could alter the amount of insulin in the dose.

Figure 5–2.9

10. Remove the needle from the bottle carefully to make sure that no insulin is lost.

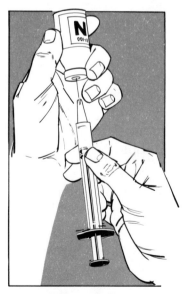

Figure 5–2.10

11. Put the syringe down, making sure that the needle does not touch anything.

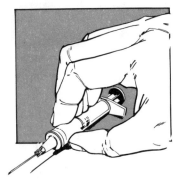

Figure 5–2.11

12a. Wipe the area you intend to inject with alcohol and a cotton swab.

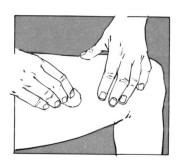

Figure 5–2.12a

12b. You can inject your insulin into the fatty tissue of the upper arms, abdomen, thighs, and buttocks. Rotate your injection sites as instructed by your physician or diabetes teaching nurse. This will prevent *lipohypertrophies* (raised toughened areas). *Lipotrophies* (deep indentations in the skin) may also occur as a result of insulin injection. They usually disappear if highly purified insulin is injected into the area of indentation. These conditions aren't permanent.

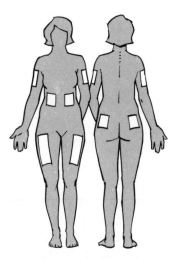

Figure 5–2.12b

13. Pinch the skin with one hand, using a good thickness of skin. When using your arm you will need someone to help you, or you can lean your arm against the wall or a door. Some authorities suggest stretching the skin taut. Fewer nerve endings are touched by the needle, and the injection may be less painful this way. Your doctor will advise the technique that is best for you.

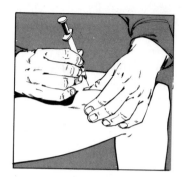

Figure 5–2.13

14. With your other hand grasp the syringe with the thumb and forefinger on the barrel and push the needle into the skin straight down.

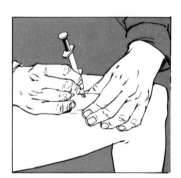

Figure 5–2.14

15. You may have been instructed to slowly pull back very slightly on the plunger before injecting the insulin, to see if any blood appears. (If this does happen, remove the needle and prepare to use a new site and syringe. The newer needles are so short that there is little likelihood of reaching a blood vessel.)

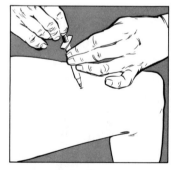

Figure 5–2.15

16. Inject the insulin by pushing down with an even pressure on the plunger.

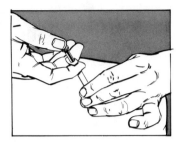

Figure 5–2.16

17. Pull the needle out of the skin. Apply pressure over the injection site with an alcohol swab. Sterilize the needle and syringe if it is the reusable type. If you are using a disposable syringe, break the needle off before discarding the syringe.

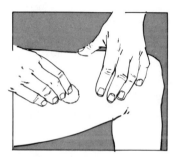

Figure 5–2.17

Two things are important to remember when giving your injection.

1. Make certain that the needle does not touch anything before you give the injection.
2. Rotate your injection sites, leaving at least an inch between injections. A still better system is to inject an arm, then a leg, then the abdomen, etc., thus insuring that you do not inject the same spot too often.

The Mixing of Insulins for Injection

To maintain better control of your diabetes, your doctor may prescribe a mixture of two types of insulin for you. While preparing this injection may seem complicated at first, the procedure can be learned quickly. You need to know the

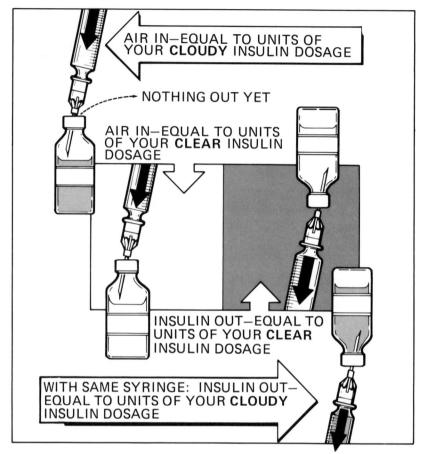

AIR IN—EQUAL TO UNITS OF YOUR **CLOUDY** INSULIN DOSAGE

NOTHING OUT YET

AIR IN—EQUAL TO UNITS OF YOUR **CLEAR** INSULIN DOSAGE

INSULIN OUT—EQUAL TO UNITS OF YOUR **CLEAR** INSULIN DOSAGE

WITH SAME SYRINGE: INSULIN OUT—EQUAL TO UNITS OF YOUR **CLOUDY** INSULIN DOSAGE

Figure 5–3. **Mixing two insulins for one injection.**

exact number of units of *each* insulin you take, and of course *both* insulins must be of the same concentration—U-100. Be sure to read the package insert of the insulins you will be using to acquaint yourself with the mixture of your prescription. This will make it very clear in your mind why you are taking a mixture instead of just a single insulin (fig. 5–3).

You will probably be mixing Regular insulin, which is clear, and one of the other longer-acting insulins, which is cloudy. Cloudy insulin is a suspension, and the bottle should be rolled gently between the palms of your hands before using it to be sure it is well mixed. Do not shake the bottle because this causes bubbles to form.

1. Prepare equipment and both insulin bottles as for a single dose. Place both bottles of insulin before you.
2. With the bottle of cloudy insulin right-side up, inject an amount of air equal to the units of the dose to be withdrawn from that bottle. Pull the needle out of the stopper without withdrawing the insulin. This puts air pressure into the bottle for later.
3. With the bottle of clear insulin right-side up, inject an amount of air equal to the number of units to be withdrawn from this vial.
4. Turn this bottle of clear insulin upside-down with the syringe still in it. Keep the end of the needle under the level of insulin in the bottle. This prevents drawing air into the syringe and cuts down on bubbles. Withdraw the specified dose.
5. With the bottle of cloudy insulin upside-down, reinsert the needle and withdraw whatever amount is required

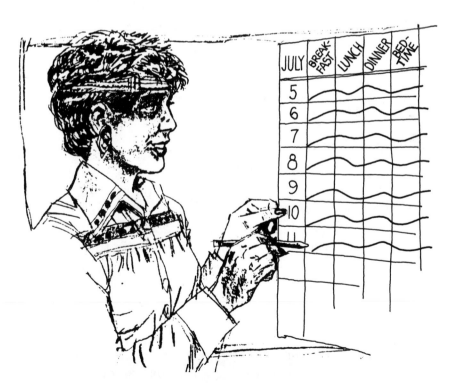

Figure 5–4. In diabetes, happiness is good control.

to make up the total units of your dose. Watch for air bubbles so that you do not push clear insulin into the cloudy insulin bottle.

6. Proceed with the injection.
7. If a mixture of two cloudy insulins, such as Lente or Semilente is prescribed, follow the same routine. The order of withdrawal makes no difference, but be sure you know the proper dose of each insulin and the total number of units of the mixed dose. It is easiest to form the habit of withdrawing the insulins in the same order every time.

Prefilling of Syringes

If you live alone and are unable to fill your syringe because of poor vision or physical disability, syringes may be prefilled by a visiting nurse or a relative and stored in the refrigerator or other cool dry place for up to 7 days. Either glass or plastic syringes may be used, and single or mixed doses of insulin may be prepared. When possible use insulins of the same brand. If a mixture is used, it is recommended that the syringe be rolled gently in the hand to mix the insulin before injecting. Keep the mixture refrigerated until the day of use.

Storage of Insulin

Insulin is very stable and does not have to be refrigerated. It will inject more comfortably at room temperature. It should, however, be protected from extremes of temperature both hot and cold. Many people keep the bottle in use at room temperature and store the reserve supplies in the refrigerator for safekeeping.

SELF-MANAGEMENT

As described earlier, diabetes is a disease in which the patient has to take responsibility for his/her own care. Self-management of diabetes by using your record of blood or urine tests as a guideline is an important step in taking full charge of your care.

1. With the advice of your doctor or health-care team, select the blood or urine tests most appropriate for you.
2. Test at the times of day directed by your doctor. Each test gives information about the action of your insulin during a different period of food intake and activity.
3. Write the results in a permanent record for future reference and note any incidents that may have affected your diabetes control, such as an emotional upset or any unplanned physical activity.
4. Review your test record at least once a week, noting any times when blood sugar was either high or low. Try to pinpoint the reasons why this occurred. If these episodes do not recur often, and your overall control is good, don't be concerned.
5. If you see a recurring pattern of high blood sugar or symptoms of reactions, contact your physician. If you have been taught self-management, change your food, activity, or insulin on your own. When adjusting your own insulin, however, be very cautious. If you have any doubts, check with your doctor before changing your dosage.
6. If your records indicate that you need to make adjustments, consider altering food first, activity second, and finally insulin.

Summary: Blood or urine tests are a "reading" of your diabetes control. Strive for as many near-to-normal tests as possible, but don't be discouraged by an occasional high blood sugar. Perfect control at all times is hard to achieve. Keep accurate records. If a recurring pattern of high or low blood sugar cannot be corrected by the methods you have been taught, consult your doctor (fig. 5–4).

6

EMERGENCIES—
BE PREPARED

INSULIN/HYPOGLYCEMIC REACTIONS

One of the most perplexing problems faced by the newly diagnosed person is the possibility of an insulin reaction (sometimes called a hypoglycemic reaction). For some people, anxiety about reactions clouds their lives and limits their normal activities. This should not be. Regardless of how well controlled diabetes is, there will be times when a reaction occurs. Knowing what to expect and what to do will help ease your fears. Learn all you can about insulin reactions, why they happen, when they may be expected, and most important, how you feel when a reaction is coming and how to treat it.

It is good to know that: (1) the majority of insulin reactions can be treated by you or your family; (2) full recovery is almost always certain; and (3) permanent ill effects from an insulin reaction only result after unconsciousness has lasted for a long period of time.

What Causes an Insulin Reaction?

An insulin reaction is caused by hypoglycemia, also known as low blood sugar. (Hypo—low, glyc—sugar, and emia—blood.) When the blood glucose level falls below 50 milligrams per 100 milliliters (fig. 6–1), a reaction may occur.

This drop in blood sugar may be caused by injection of too much insulin, too much exercise, too little food, or by drinking alcohol without eating any food.

What's Going On?

The most upsetting part of an insulin reaction is that it usually happens so fast. You are feeling good, working hard, or perhaps exercising and suddenly you begin to tremble, the palms of your hands perspire, you feel nervous and hungry, your heart begins to pound, and your breath comes faster. You may also experience only a sense of vague uneasiness, a headache, or slight nausea.

For example, suppose you are a homemaker dusting a windowsill and notice that the window is very dirty. You decide to wash it and then discover that several others need

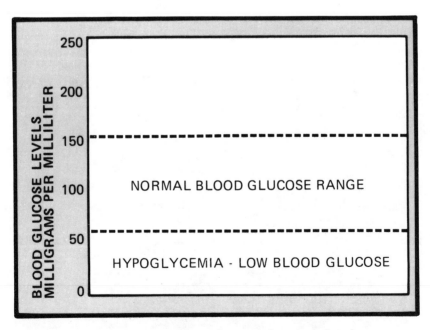

Figure 6–1. **Blood glucose (sugar) ranges for normal and hypoglycemic levels.**

attention, so you go ahead and wash them all. Such unplan-ned activity could cause a reaction. Or maybe you are a teenager riding your bike home from school. You usually have a snack when you get home. But it is such a glorious day you decide to take a detour which adds extra miles to your regular ride. Pedaling home an hour or so later you suddenly feel shaky. The added exercise has lowered your blood sugar below normal limits (fig. 6–2).

Treatment at this point is vital to prevent the reaction from getting worse. When untreated, the symptoms become more marked, but the victim is less aware of what is happen-ing. Those around you may notice that you've suddenly be-come pale, irritable, quarrelsome, your conversation doesn't make much sense, your body movements are jerky, and you may have difficulty walking. If untreated, a reaction can progress to temporary unconsciousness, but this is not usual and can be prevented.

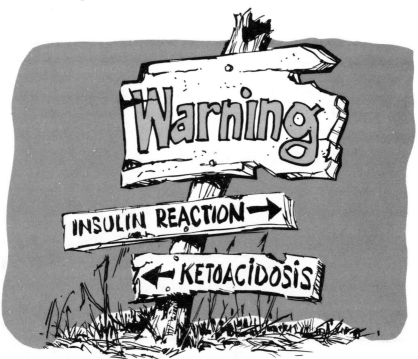

Figure 6–2. Watch for the signs.

The treatment for an insulin reaction is *sugar* in any form, taken at the first sign of a reaction. This can be sugar cubes, candy such as lifesavers, orange juice, a nondiet soda, a tablespoon of honey, corn syrup, or one of the forms of quick glucose that is sold specifically for insulin reactions. If, after 10 to 15 minutes, your symptoms still persist, repeat the treatment. When you feel better, eat some protein food such as a cheese or a meat sandwich and a glass of milk. This will help keep your blood-sugar level up.

Glucagon

If unconsciousness does occur and the person is unable to swallow, an injection of glucagon should be given immediately. Glucagon is a hormone that raises blood sugar. It is available only by prescription. Ask your doctor to prescribe it for you. Every insulin-dependent person should keep glucagon at home and at work. Make certain that someone in the family and a coworker knows how to inject it should the need arise. An insulin syringe is used for injecting glucagon.

General Directions for Use

- Glucagon is an emergency drug to be used only under the direction of a physician. Become familiar with the following instructions before the emergency arises.
- In case of insulin coma or severe reactions, administer glucagon and call a physician promptly.
- Act quickly. Unconsciousness over a period of time may be very harmful.
- Inject glucagon in the same way that insulin is injected (see the following directions). Turn patient to one side or face down. Rest face on arms.
- The patient usually awakens within 15 minutes. Feed the patient as soon as he awakens.
- Glucagon is a safe drug. There is no danger of overdosage.

Note: Glucagon should not be prepared for injection until the emergency arises.

Follow the step-by-step procedure outlined below for mixing and preparing the injection.

To Prepare Glucagon for Injection
(Reprinted with permission of Eli Lilly Company and the American Diabetes Association.)

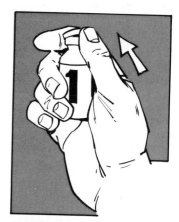

1. Remove the flip-off seals on bottles Nos. 1 and 2.

2. Wipe the rubber stoppers on both bottles with a suitable antiseptic if available (alcohol or isopropyl alcohol).

3. Use a U-40 or U-100 insulin syringe and needle.

Figure 6–3.1

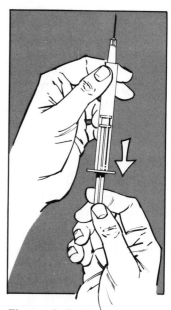

4. Draw the plunger of the syringe back to the 20-unit mark on a U-40 syringe or to the 50-unit mark on a U-100 syringe.

Figure 6–3.2

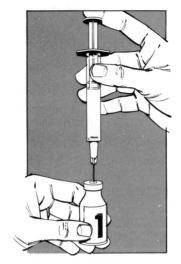

5. Pick up the smaller, white-labeled bottle (No. 1) containing the diluting solution. Pierce the center of the stopper with the needle attached to the syringe.

Figure 6–3.3

6. Turn the bottle upside-down and inject the air from the syringe into the bottle. It will then be possible to remove the diluting solution more easily.

7. Keep the tip of the needle in the diluting solution and withdraw as much of the solution as possible into the syringe.

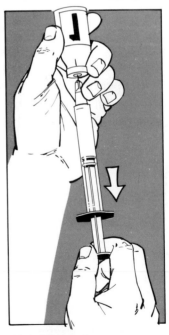

Figure 6–3.4

8. Remove the needle and syringe from bottle No. 1 and insert this same needle into the bottle (No. 2) containing the glucagon. Inject all of the diluting solution from the syringe into bottle No. 2.

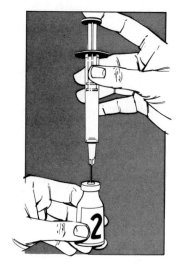

Figure 6–3.5

9. Remove needle and syringe. Shake bottle gently. The glucagon will dissolve, and the preparation will become clear. Withdraw the entire contents of the bottle into the syringe. The solution is now ready for injection into the patient.

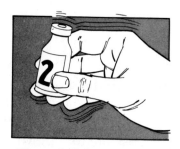

Figure 6–3.6

To Administer Glucagon
(Note: This is the same technique as for injecting insulin.)

1. Select the injection site. Glucagon is administered like insulin. It can be given in the abdomen, buttocks, upper and outer thigh, or the back, fatty part of the upper arm.

2. Wipe the site with cotton dipped in alcohol.

3. Pinch up the area of skin and fat to be injected.

4. Inject needle through skin. (A 90° angle is satisfactory unless the diabetic is extremely thin. In that case, use a 45° angle.)

5. Push on plunger to inject the entire amount of glucagon. (If the person being treated is under three years old, use only half the dose.)

6. Withdraw the needle from the skin.

7. Press the cotton gently on the injection site.

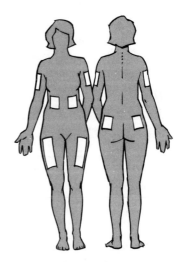

Figure 6–3.7

When treated with glucagon, the severe hypoglycemic state usually subsides, and the person awakens within 15 minutes. If the unconscious person vomits as he is waking up, he should be turned face down or on one side to help prevent breathing any stomach contents into his lungs.

As soon as the patient is alert enough to swallow, feed him some carbohydrate! (Examples of quick carbohydrate sources include soft drinks, orange juice, and sugar dissolved in water.) This should be followed by a longer-acting carbohydrate, such as a cracker or a sandwich, to avoid a second hypoglycemic episode, since glucagon acts for only a short period of time.

Other Instructions: If the unconscious person does not awaken within 20 minutes, the dose may be repeated, and a physician should be consulted as soon as possible.

If you find the person unconscious and are not sure whether his comatose condition is due to high (hyper-) or low (hypo-) blood sugar, it is best to assume this is a low (hypo-) blood sugar state and to give glucagon.

Do not use the glucagon after the date stamped on the label of bottle No. 2.

How Supplied: Glucagon is available in two forms: an emergency kit with one vial containing the purified glucagon in dry powder form and a syringe prefilled with a diluting solution; and a two-bottle package with one bottle containing the purified glucagon in dry powder form and the other containing a diluting solution.

Where Available: Glucagon is a prescription drug available at most pharmacies. The cost varies from one drugstore to another. Ask your doctor to prescribe it for you.

Your Responsibility

When you have diabetes you have the primary responsibility for preventing and treating an insulin reaction. Always carry some form of sugar with you and take this at the first feeling of a reaction. Always wear some type of identification, either a bracelet or neck chain which says, "I have diabetes." Always carry an identification card in your wallet or purse, so that should you be confused during a reaction, someone could recognize your condition and help you promptly. In the home, at school, at work, at sporting events, or when traveling, make certain that those around you know that you have diabetes and what to do in case of a reaction. Prevent a reaction whenever possible. Treat a reaction quickly when one occurs. Don't be embarrassed by a reaction. Resume your activity as soon as you feel better.

Try to Remember

After you have had a reaction try to remember what you were doing at the time that might have caused it. Think carefully about how you felt. Everyone is unique, and feelings during a reaction can be different from person to person. Remembering how you felt will help you recognize an oncoming reaction in the future. Make notes on the episode for your doctor. This will help pinpoint the causes. Try to avoid situations that might cause a reaction. Anticipate the effects of a late meal by eating something beforehand; for example, if you are invited out for dinner and don't know whether it will be served at your usual hour or later, eat one Bread Exchange from your dinner meal plan before you go and then pass up something equal to one Bread Exchange when dinner is served. Allow for unplanned activity or exercise by eating a snack beforehand (see chapter 3).

Be Prepared

Always carry some form of sugar with you—sugar cubes, candy, or one of the forms of quick glucose. There are commercial products available which come in a small tube and can be squeezed into the mouth between teeth and cheek for quick absorption. These are handy to carry and not so tasty that they are tempting to use when you don't need them. On days when you are planning a strenuous activity, carry an extra sandwich, crackers and cheese, or peanut butter.

An Ounce of Prevention

Prevention is the key word for reactions, insofar as this is possible. When you take your insulin in the morning, keep in mind that it is inside your body doing its job, lowering your blood sugar for eight hours or longer. If you don't eat on time, or don't eat all the food your meal plan calls for, a reaction will occur.

Points to Remember

1. Always eat your meals and snacks on time. This is just as important as taking your insulin.
2. Eat everything your meal plan calls for. Your insulin is prescribed to match the amount of food you eat. If you don't eat all the food in your plan, you may upset your diabetes control.
3. Always carry some form of sugar for treating a reaction.
4. Always eat before exercising.
5. Don't drink alcohol without eating some food.

Do All People with Diabetes Have Insulin Reactions?

Reactions usually occur in people who take insulin. Persons who take oral drugs to control their diabetes may have a reaction, but this is not usual. Reactions do not occur in persons who control their diabetes with diet alone.

Summary: The causes of hypoglycemia/insulin reaction are: too much insulin, too much exercise, too little food, drinking alcohol without eating some food.

The symptoms are: abrupt or sudden shaking or trembling, faintness, blurred vision, headache, numbness in the arms and hands, a tingling sensation around the mouth, hunger, a pounding heart, inability to think clearly, sudden and unexplained irritability or hostility, skin pallor, a vacant staring or dazed expression, and clumsy or jerky movements, especially when walking.

The treatment is: take some form of sugar at the first sign of a reaction. If no relief is felt within 15 minutes, repeat this treatment. When the symptoms have passed eat some protein food. Resume your exercise or activity as soon as you feel better.

If unconsciousness occurs, an injection of glucagon should be given immediately. If no improvement is visible within 15 minutes call the doctor or take the person to the nearest hospital for emergency treatment.

THE SOMOGYI EFFECT

The Somogyi effect is the result of mixed body signals. It can be likened to a faulty thermostat that doesn't shut off when the desired temperature is reached. The body signals indicate that more insulin is needed, when actually just the opposite is true.

In treating persons with hard-to-control diabetes, Dr. Somogyi found some years ago that if too much insulin is given, it causes a prolonged insulin reaction without any apparent symptoms. For example, when a reaction occurs at night it can go unnoticed. When blood sugar falls below normal, the body releases hormones to raise it, such as adrenalin, glucagon, growth hormones, and cortisone. This causes the next test to be high in sugar. Adrenalin also causes a breakdown of fat in the body and produces ketones in the urine. The combination of high blood sugar and ketones in the urine makes it appear that there is a need for more insulin, when less insulin is what is actually needed.

If the insulin dose is increased when the urine shows high levels of sugar and ketones, the blood sugar will be temporarily lowered, then the released hormones will cause it to rise to an even higher level than before. Because all of the insulin injected is never completely used, a cycle or rebound effect is created, and swings from high to low blood sugar are repeated over and over.

The possibility of a Somogyi effect should be suspected when:

1. The total dose of insulin per day exceeds ½ unit per pound of body weight. A person's need varies, but this is a general rule.
2. Morning urine tests are high in sugar and ketones.
3. Increasing the dose of insulin does not bring blood sugar levels down.
4. A low morning temperature is evident. An insulin reaction causes a drop in temperature for approximately five to six hours. If a reaction occurs during the night, the temperature could be low upon awakening.
5. Morning headache occurs.

Because of the swings from low to high blood sugar, the Somogyi effect has an impact on the emotions. You may experience irritability, depression, and a general feeling of fatigue, or being "out of sorts."

The Treatment

When the Somogyi effect is suspected it requires professional treatment. Your doctor will adjust your insulin dose and possibly redistribute your food and activity throughout the day, in order to achieve better glucose control with the least amount of insulin. You need to know the symptoms and recognize them if they do occur, so that you can call them to your doctor's attention.

KETOACIDOSIS/DIABETIC COMA

There is a great deal of confusion about the terms *insulin reaction* and *diabetic coma*. An insulin reaction is a sudden and unexpected emergency that usually happens in minutes and is caused by hypoglycemia, lower than normal blood sugar. A diabetic coma is also an emergency, but it develops more slowly, over a period of hours or even days, and is caused by hyperglycemia, higher than normal blood sugar. The causes, symptoms, and treatment for these two conditions are different. As a diabetic person, it is important for you to know the signs of both conditions. Figure 6–4 shows the symptoms of insulin reaction and diabetic coma side by side so that you can fix them in your mind. (Keep the chart handy, since with either condition you're not fully alert.)

What Causes a Diabetic Coma?

A coma occurs when diabetes gets out of control and blood sugar rises to dangerous levels. When there is too much glucose in the blood and not enough insulin, the glucose/ sugar cannot enter the cells. The body then must use its reserves of proteins and fat to burn for energy. This causes ketones to appear in the urine in large amounts. The presence of high blood sugar and ketones in the urine should always be a cause of concern to the person with diabetes and should be reported to the doctor promptly. When ketones and glucose are found, and more insulin is prescribed promptly, development of ketoacidosis is prevented.

The causes of hyperglycemia (high blood sugar) leading to ketoacidosis and coma are infection or illness, neglect in taking insulin or taking too small a dose, overeating, or a combination of these factors.

The early symptoms of thirst, frequent urination, and large amounts of glucose and ketones in the urine are significant. Other symptoms appear gradually: the skin becomes flushed and dry, the person is drowsy, the breath has a fruity odor, breathing is labored, vomiting and abdominal pain are present. When these symptoms are found, the doctor should be notified promptly. Treatment for ketoacidosis must take place in the hospital and consists of insulin administration and close monitoring of blood glucose over a period of time in order to bring the diabetes under control.

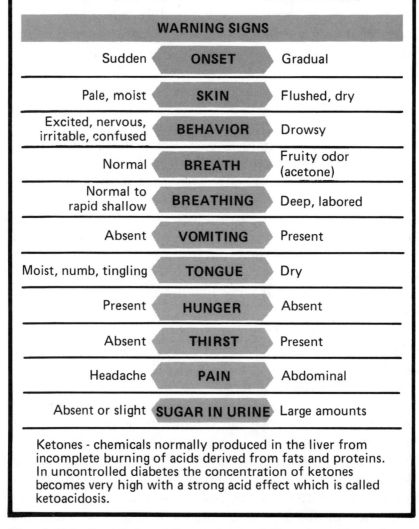

HOW CAN YOU TELL WHICH REACTION IS TAKING PLACE?

The following warning signals will quickly identify the reaction and indicate the proper treatment:

HYPOGLYCEMIC REACTION (Insulin Reaction)		KETOACIDOSIS (Diabetic Coma)
	WARNING SIGNS	
Sudden	**ONSET**	Gradual
Pale, moist	**SKIN**	Flushed, dry
Excited, nervous, irritable, confused	**BEHAVIOR**	Drowsy
Normal	**BREATH**	Fruity odor (acetone)
Normal to rapid shallow	**BREATHING**	Deep, labored
Absent	**VOMITING**	Present
Moist, numb, tingling	**TONGUE**	Dry
Present	**HUNGER**	Absent
Absent	**THIRST**	Present
Headache	**PAIN**	Abdominal
Absent or slight	**SUGAR IN URINE**	Large amounts

Ketones - chemicals normally produced in the liver from incomplete burning of acids derived from fats and proteins. In uncontrolled diabetes the concentration of ketones becomes very high with a strong acid effect which is called ketoacidosis.

Figure 6–4. Comparison of symptoms of hypoglycemia and hyperglycemia. (Reprinted from "What You Need to Know About Diabetes." American Diabetes Association, Inc.)

Ketoacidosis/diabetic coma usually occurs in the ketosis-prone insulin-dependent Type I person. It does not occur in Type II people. It can also happen to a person who has diabetes but does not know it. Diabetic coma is fairly uncommon today. It is important, however, to know the symptoms and to report them to your doctor promptly should they occur.

Summary: All people with diabetes should be aware of the signs of hyperglycemia: high blood sugar, ketones in the urine, extreme thirst, and drowsiness. Knowing how you feel when your blood sugar is higher than normal will help you avoid serious emergencies.

HYPEROSMOLAR NONKETOTIC COMA

This is a diabetic emergency found most often in elderly persons with diabetes. It can also occur in older persons with no previous diagnosis of diabetes. In this type of coma ketones are not found in the urine, hence the term *nonketotic*.

The word *hyperosmolar* indicates an upset in the concentration of chemicals in the various body fluids. As hyperosmolar coma develops, the blood sugar builds up over a period of days to very high levels. As the blood sugar increases, it causes water to be drawn from the cells and from extracellular spaces in the tissues. The extra volume of fluid is passed off in the urine with the glucose, causing great thirst, weakness, and serious dehydration.

Hyperosmolar coma is caused by some event that increases the body's need for insulin, such as an acute illness, stroke, infection, accident, physical or emotional stress, or from eating large amounts of concentrated sugars. It can also be caused by large doses of drugs such as steroids, diuretics, or tranquilizers, and poor kidney function.

The *symptoms* include extreme weakness, fatigue, high blood or urine sugars, excessive thirst, dehydration, dry mouth, shallow breathing, flushed dry skin, mental confusion, drowsiness, and finally stupor and coma.

Hyperosmolar coma always requires treatment in the hospital. Insulin is given, lost fluids are replaced, and blood glucose levels are monitored closely. Family members of the elderly diabetic person should know the signs of developing hyperglycemia, which can lead to hyperosmolar coma. This condition is life-threatening, and early recognition and prompt treatment are of the utmost importance.

7 TYPE II NON-INSULIN-DEPENDENT DIABETES

Of the two main types of diabetes, Type II is the more easily controlled. In fact, some doctors are now saying that this type of diabetes can be "cured" if caught early and treated successfully. Since the majority of people in this category are overweight at the time of diagnosis, weight loss is the first choice of treatment. When excess weight is lost, and the loss maintained, the symptoms almost always disappear, and blood sugar remains within normal limits. The symptoms and the diabetes will reappear, however, if the weight is regained.

The treatment of the obese person with Type II diabetes consists of reducing body weight to a desirable level and maintaining the weight loss with a prescribed daily meal plan restricted in calories.

How Obesity Affects Diabetes

The pancreas has approximately 100,000 islets of Langerhans, clusters of cells each of which contains 80 to 100 beta cells. These are the cells that make up the insulin factory of the body. After a meal is consumed, the pancreas receives a signal to release an amount of insulin sufficient to balance the glucose produced during digestion. The more food taken into the body, the more insulin required and released into the bloodstream. Diabetic people who are overweight usually have enough insulin; sometimes they have an excess (hyperinsulinism), but it is not used effectively because of a lack of insulin-binding cell receptors.

A cell receptor is an acutely sensitive area on the cell that attracts insulin as it circulates in the blood. As the receptor grasps the insulin it combines with blood glucose and enters the cell to be used in energy production. Progressive obesity seems to diminish the number of cell receptors. So although the beta cells in the overweight person may be producing a sufficient amount of insulin and releasing it into the bloodstream, if there are too few receptors working properly, there is no way for the glucose to enter the cells.

Research has shown that the lack of functioning insulin-binding receptors in the overweight person is reversible. As weight is lost, the receptors become active again. Glucose is able to enter the cells and blood glucose is lowered.

Other factors related to body weight may also be involved in adult-onset diabetes. It is believed that over a period of time, perhaps even years, the extra demands on the pancreas created by excess weight cause the beta cells to lose their insulin-producing ability and eventually stop altogether. This too, is reversed when weight is lost.

WHAT IS OBESITY?

Obesity is the condition of being overweight. A person is said to be obese when body weight exceeds 20 percent of normal (see table 7–1). Obesity is a lifelong disease. The tendency to it appears to run in families. The causes are thought to include socioeconomic, ethnic, cultural, and psychological factors. Recent studies about an enzyme called ATPase may provide some further answers to the puzzling question of obesity. (An enzyme is a protein produced by living cells which reacts chemically in a variety of body processes, including digestion.) Why can some people eat all they want and stay slim, and others need only to look at a gourmet menu to gain weight? An error in body chemistry that was first found in mice in laboratory tests has been discovered in humans. This error in metabolism may indicate why some people have trouble controlling their weight. In a study of the levels of ATPase in twenty-three obese subjects, blood samples were compared with those of individuals at normal weight. The levels of ATPase were significantly lower in the twenty-three obese subjects, and the heavier the person the lower the ATPase level.

ATPase is essential to the body in forcing sodium and potassium, chemicals necessary for normal body functioning, across cell membranes. The heat generated in this process uses considerable calories, and normally represents anywhere from 10 to 50 percent of the body's total heat production. From the study it appears that low levels of ATPase may predispose people to being overweight because fewer calories than normal are burned for energy, and more calories are stored as fat in the body. The results of this study may lead to new ways of treating obesity in the future.

TABLE 7–1
TABLE FOR COMPUTING DESIRABLE BODY WEIGHT

Women	100 pounds for the first 5 feet of height plus 5 pounds for each additional inch (plus 10 percent for a large frame, and minus 10 percent for a small frame).
Men	106 pounds for the first 5 feet of height plus 6 pounds for each additional inch (plus 10 percent for a large frame and minus 10 percent for a small frame).

Can Obesity Be Controlled?

Controlling weight is a lifelong struggle for many people. A few years ago Daniel B. Stone, M.D. provided the following formula and suggested that all people who are overweight keep it foremost in their minds:

Calories in, equal to calories out = weight unchanged
Calories in, greater than calories out = weight gain
Calories in, less than calories out = weight loss

Weight loss results when more calories are burned than are consumed. Excess weight cannot be lost overnight; it must be a gradual process. Weight is gained gradually by most people, and it can creep up unnoticed.

For example, if a person eats just one more slice of bread per day than is needed, the calories-in exceeding the calories-out will be 70 per day. This translates into an annual weight gain of 7.3 pounds per year. Over a period of 10 years this adds up to a hefty 70 pounds (fig. 7–1).

THE DIET PRESCRIPTION

Your physician or dietitian will prescribe a daily meal plan for you that meets your nutritional needs, by taking into consideration your work, your physical activity, including any newly prescribed exercise plan if necessary, and your general lifestyle. It will be sufficiently restricted in calories to enable you to lose weight gradually. Naturally, everyone has different caloric needs. For example, an overweight laborer will need more calories each day than a housewife engaged in semisedentary work.

A diet history will be taken to determine the background of the obesity: eating habits, socioeconomic status, knowledge of nutrition, and reasons for previous failures to lose weight. The best plan is to achieve a weight loss of two pounds per week. This may not always be possible, but it should be your aim. Your health professional will tell you the total amount of weight you need to lose and how to go about it. The rest is up to you. Diabetes is a life-threatening disease if it is not controlled. Type II diabetes can frequently be controlled with diet. You will have to count calories and possibly become more knowledgeable about nutrition.

Here are some tips to help you in your weight-loss program.

1. Keep a food diary for a week. This will show you when and why you are likely to overeat. Were you

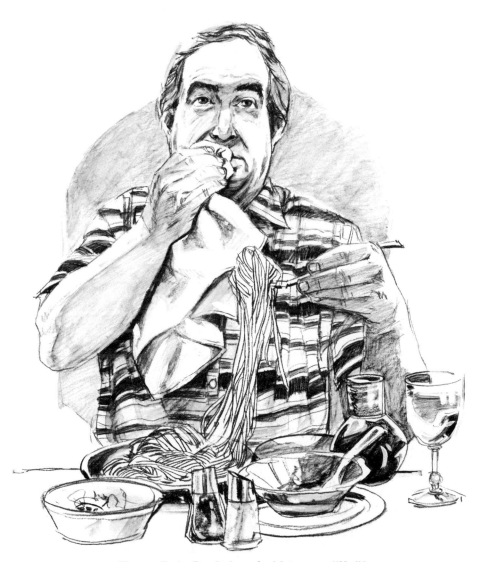

Figure 7–1. **Don't be afraid to say "No"!**

angry, bored, or watching someone on TV who was snacking? Knowing the reasons will help you to change your behavior.

2. To be effective, weight reduction should be gradual. Don't expect miracles. By following your diet pre-

scription conscientiously, one day at a time, you will soon notice the numbers on your scale dropping.

3. Eat slowly. Chew each mouthful 20 times before swallowing. The stomach takes 20 to 30 minutes to signal the brain that it is full. If you eat too fast, the signal to stop goes unnoticed.

4. If you are the food shopper in your house, make a list and stick to it. Never go to the supermarket when you are hungry. This will only tempt you to buy things you shouldn't have and don't need.

5. Brushing the teeth after a meal will rid your mouth of the taste of food.

6. Never skip a meal; it will only cause you to overeat at the next meal.

7. If you cook and serve the meals at your house, trim recipes so there aren't too many leftovers. Reject second portions and get someone else to clean up and wash the dishes. This way you won't be tempted to nibble the leftovers.

8. Learn how to avoid forbidden foods at social functions, or stay away until you have lost some weight and gained some willpower.

9. When you are tempted to nibble, take a walk, pursue a hobby, or learn a new skill; do anything to take your mind away from food.

10. Exercise will help, and contrary to some opinion it does not increase appetite.

11. Enlist the help of your spouse and your family in your diet program. Family support of the person who needs to lose weight is important psychologically.

A portly cellist, member of a large symphony orchestra, when told by his doctor that he had diabetes and would have to lose some weight, became quite indignant.

"I don't have time for diabetes and dieting," he protested. "My schedule is filled, my hours long, there are rehearsals, performances, and travel! How can I follow a diet?"

Finally the doctor interrupted him, "Doesn't you wife have diabetes?"

"Yes, she's had it for years," admitted the portly patient, "only I never paid much attention to how she handles it." When he and his wife worked on their common problem, he was able to bring his weight down and control his diabetes and still keep his busy schedule.

EXERCISE AND WEIGHT CONTROL

All of the benefits of exercise have been described in chapter 3. It should be emphasized, however, that exercise is essential for the overweight person as an adjunct to a calorie-controlled diet. Before beginning an exercise program, check with your doctor, particularly if you haven't exercised for some time.

Make little things count. Climb stairs instead of taking an elevator or escalator. Walk when you can instead of taking your car. This will use your energy and save the world's for future generations. Walking is the best, safest, and easiest exercise, and it can be done with ease on a regular basis. Calisthenics are excellent if you like them and when done to music become even more enjoyable.

Any physical activity performed at least two or three times a week is beneficial; it improves circulation, trims the figure, provides a sense of well-being, and helps control diabetes.

ORAL DRUGS

What Are Oral Hypoglycemic Compounds?

These are drugs taken by mouth that stimulate the release of insulin in the body. In order for these drugs to be effective, the pancreas must be able to produce *some* insulin; therefore, they can only be used in the treatment of Type II diabetes. These drugs are *not* oral insulin as is sometimes thought. (Insulin is a protein and cannot be taken by mouth because it is destroyed by the stomach's digestive juices.) These drugs are *not* a substitute for a diet and are *only effective* in the overweight patient when used with a calorie-restricted meal plan. Oral drugs are known by the trade names Acetohexamide (Dymelor®), Chlorpropamide (Diabinese®), Tolazamide (Tolinase), Tolbutamide (Orinase®), Glyburide (DiaBeta®, Micronase®), and Glipizide (Glucatrol®), and they come in tablet form. Each oral drug has a particular action time, and if you take one of these drugs you should know what this is (see table 7–2).

INTERACTION WITH OTHER DRUGS

Persons who take oral hypoglycemic agents should be aware that some prescription drugs, as well as alcoholic beverages, can interact infavorably with oral hypoglycemic agents. If your physician prescribes an oral drug to control your diabetes, remind him/her of any other medications you are taking. If you use alcohol discuss this also.

TABLE 7–2
ORAL HYPOGLYCEMIC AGENTS

Drug	Comparative Dose (mg)	Usual Minimum and Maximum Daily Dose	Duration of Activity
First-generation sulfonylureas Acetohexamide (Dymelor)	500	0.25–1.5 gm single or divided doses	12–18 plus hrs.
Chlorpropamide (Diabinese)	250	0.1–0.5 gm single dose	24–72 hrs.
Tolazamide (Tolinase)	250	0.1–1.0 gm single or divided doses	10–16 plus hrs.
Tolbutamide (Orinase)	1,000	0.5–2.0 gm divided doses	6–12 hrs.
Second-generation sulfonylureas Glyburide (DiaBeta) (Micronase)	5	1.25–20 mg single or divided doses	24 hrs.
Glipizide (Glucotrol)	5	2.5–40 mg single or divided doses	16–24 hrs.

Source: Adapted from and printed with permission of R. Keith Campbell, R.Ph., MBA.

Before you take an over-the-counter drug (medicine that can be bought without a prescription) be sure to read the label. You may have sometimes noticed a warning, "Not to be taken by persons who have diabetes." Liquid cold medicines and cough depressants often contain large amounts of sugar and alcohol, both of which add calories. Medicines for colds, allergies, and asthma may also raise blood pressure and cause constriction of the small blood vessels. Doctors generally suggest this basic rule: avoid nonprescription drugs unless they are actually needed. Rather than risk the side effects and jeopardize your diabetes control, it is sometimes better to put up with such symptoms as a stuffy head or a slight cough.

When Is Insulin Used in Type II Diabetes?

As noted earlier, when diet fails, insulin or oral drugs will be added to the treatment program. Insulin may be prescribed after a diet has been thoroughly tried. It is often necessary to use insulin temporarily during serious illness or surgery.

Summary: For the overweight diabetic person the preferred treatment for Type II diabetes is diet. This diet must be individually prescribed, provide the patient with enough carbohydrates, proteins, and fats to maintain good nutrition, and be limited in total calories to enable the person to lose excess weight and maintain the loss.

For the 10 percent of Type II diabetic people who are not overweight, the diet should be individually prescribed allowing for optimal nutrition, sufficient calories to maintain ideal body weight, and adequate control of diabetes.

8

PROBLEMS— COMPLICATIONS

There are two general types of blood vessel (vascular) disease that occur in persons with diabetes: *microangiopathy* and *macroangiopathy* or small and large vessel disease (micro—small, macro—large, angio—vessel, and pathy—disease).

Microangiopathy only occurs in persons with diabetes. Although it has been found in almost every organ of the body in persons with diabetes, it usually occurs in the retina of the eye (the camera that produces the pictures) and the glomeruli of the kidneys (the tiny capillaries that filter wastes from the blood to form urine). See the sections on retinopathy and nephropathy for more detailed information.

What happens to the small blood vessels? In the person with diabetes, the inner lining of the walls of small blood vessels, known as the basement membranes, become thickened, reducing the size of the channel through which the blood flows. When the organs nourished by the small blood vessels, especially the eyes and the kidneys, are deprived of an adequate blood supply, they lose some of their function.

Why this occurs only in persons with diabetes is not fully understood. It is thought that the basement membranes are affected by the abnormal swings in blood sugar that occur in diabetes and that this deprives the tissues of essential chemicals needed for growth and replacement, causing the membranes to thicken and the blood vessels to narrow.

Can Microangiopathy Be Prevented?

No one knows for sure, but there is some proof that strict control of diabetes may delay the onset of small blood vessel disease. And there are some diabetologists (doctors who specialize in treating diabetes) who now think that the course of the disease may be stopped and possibly even turned around when blood sugar levels are kept as close to normal as possible at all times.

Macroangiopathy, large vessel disease, is the other type of vascular disease to which diabetic people are prone. Normally, blood vessels undergo changes due to age, high blood pressure, obesity, smoking, a diet high in fat, and stress. The changes that occur in the large blood vessels of the diabetic person are no different than those in the nondiabetic. They tend to appear sooner, however, and often are more severe.

Arteriosclerosis is the most common cause of large blood vessel disease. It affects the major arteries which carry blood to the arms, legs, head, lungs, and abdominal organs. The arteries of the body can be likened to the trunk and main branches of a tree, the small blood vessels to the many smaller branches which reach out to nourish the leaves. Keeping this in mind it is easy to see that when the arteries are affected by arteriosclerosis, the flow of blood into the small blood vessels is decreased, and the body parts fed by these vessels are deprived of needed nourishment.

In arteriosclerosis the blood vessels become thick and rigid (lose their elasticity), and the inner lining of the walls becomes spotted with calcium and fatlike patches. While arteriosclerosis can cause a decreased flow of blood to the heart, the brain, and the kidneys, persons with diabetes are most often affected in the legs and feet.

How Are the Legs and Feet Affected?

As arteriosclerosis develops, the blood vessels become narrowed, and the blood supply is reduced, particularly to the legs and feet. This causes cramping, weakness, and pain in the calves of the legs when walking. When the leg is rested the pain goes away. The pain is present because the narrowed artery is unable to supply enough blood and oxygen to the muscles during exercise.

When ischemia (inadequate blood supply) is suspected, the physician will look for other signs. The skin on the affected leg may be shiny, cool, and hairless. When the leg is raised, the skin pales rapidly, and when it is dangled, the foot and the toes will have a bluish, red color. The toenails may be brittle, there may be a loss of pulse in the groin, behind the knee, and in the foot. Small cracks in the skin, particularly on the soles of the feet, may be another sign of an inadequate blood supply.

The exact location of the blocked artery can be found either by tracing the path of the artery with an electronic instrument that "beeps" when passed over a blocked artery or by taking an angiogram. An angiogram is an X ray of the arteries made after a dye is injected into the main artery above the suspected trouble site (fig. 8–1). This helps the doctor to see the exact extent of the damage in the vessel and where the blockage occurs.

What Is the Treatment?

Repair of a blocked blood vessel using a surgical "bypass" can be highly successful. In this surgery either a new vein is made from one taken from the patient or a dacron tube is inserted above and below the diseased portion of the artery, making a detour around the blocked portion. It should be noted, however, that while this surgery is successful in 70 percent of cases and corrects the blocked blood vessel, it does not correct the cause of arteriosclerosis. Strict attention to

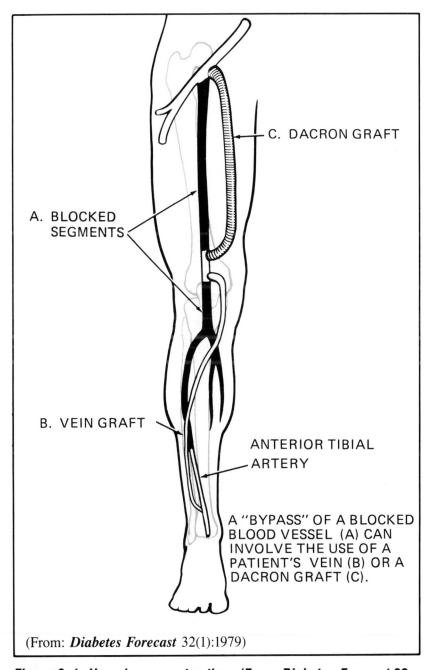

C. DACRON GRAFT

A. BLOCKED
SEGMENTS

B. VEIN GRAFT

ANTERIOR TIBIAL
ARTERY

A "BYPASS" OF A BLOCKED
BLOOD VESSEL (A) CAN
INVOLVE THE USE OF A
PATIENT'S VEIN (B) OR A
DACRON GRAFT (C).

(From: *Diabetes Forecast* 32(1):1979)

Figure 8–1. Vascular reconstruction. (From *Diabetes Forecast* 32 [1]: 1979)

diet, blood glucose control, and elimination of smoking are absolutely necessary to prevent a recurrence.

Gangrene and Amputation

Gangrene is a serious complication of diabetes. However, it can often be prevented if the symptoms leading to the condition are observed and treated promptly. When the blood supply to a tissue is cut off for six or more hours, the tissue becomes numb and dark-colored and dies. Death of a tissue is called gangrene. Although amputation due to gangrene is sometimes necessary to save the rest of the limb, this complication of diabetes has decreased remarkably in the past 20 years as a result of improved methods of treatment and patient awareness of problems or injuries that could lead to gangrene.

Prevention of blood vessel disease should be the aim of every diabetic person. Be aware of the symptoms of vascular disease and see your doctor at the first sign of trouble. Although aging causes some wear and tear on the blood vessels, it is very important for anyone with diabetes to observe the rules of good foot care. Daily exercise, particularly walking, is helpful in preventing or delaying large blood vessel disease.

Summary: Strict control of blood glucose appears to be the diabetic's best insurance against vascular disease. Following are some guidelines believed to delay the onset, slow the progress, and possibly even reverse vascular disease in diabetes.

1. If you smoke, STOP. This is of the utmost importance.
2. Keep blood glucose under good control.
3. Eat nutritious, well-balanced meals, with special attention to a reduction of fats.
4. Maintain normal body weight.
5. Exercise regularly.
6. Control high blood pressure.

VISUAL PROBLEMS

The eye is one of the body's major miracles. Light enters through the cornea, the transparent outer covering, and is focused by the lens on the retina. The light-sensitive cells of the retina send signals to the brain by way of the optic nerves. The brain receives the image and "explains" what is seen. From the time we open our eyes in the morning until we close them at night, the eye is sending messages to the brain without any conscious effort on our part (fig. 8–2).

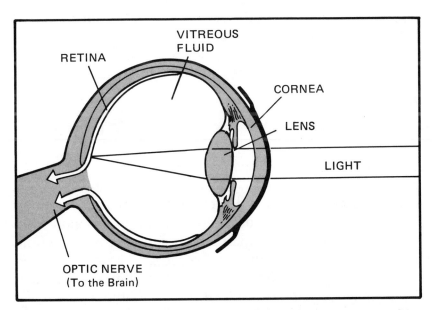

Figure 8–2. **Cross section of the eye. (From *Diabetes Forecast* 31 [6]: 1978)**

Minor Eye Problems in Diabetes

There are several minor eye problems that sometimes cause unnecessary worry, especially to newly diagnosed people. Blurred vision is one of these. When diabetes is first discovered, this may be a problem that can last several weeks until the diabetes is brought under control. Prolonged high blood sugar can cause a loss of fluid within the eye, and the shifting fluid in turn can also cause blurred vision.

Double vision sometimes occurs. This may be caused by low blood sugar or by the nerves that control the eye muscles when these are affected by neuropathy, a disease of the nerves. This is a disturbing problem, but it is important to know that this usually improves as blood sugar is brought under control (see the section on neuropathy).

Hemorrhage of the conjunctiva, the outer lining of the eye, occurs when a blood vessel ruptures. This does not disturb vision and is not serious. It can be caused by rubbing or other irritations, or for no known reason. All three of these conditions are usually minor and temporary and will clear up within a short period of time.

Diabetic Retinopathy

While blindness is a cause of great concern to all diabetic people, it is important to know that contrary to popular opinion, the vast majority of people with diabetes do not develop severe diabetic retinopathy, disease of the retina.

There are two types of diabetic retinopathy: background, which affects the inside of the retina and is the more common, and proliferative, which affects the vitreous (the fluid-filled chamber in the center of the eye).

Background retinopathy is caused by changes that occur in the capillaries, the small blood vessels that join the arteries and the veins. Microaneurysms, tiny bulges containing fluid and fatty particles, develop and tend to block the flow of blood (fig. 8–3). These bulges break easily, leaking fluid and blood inside the retina. Some microaneurysms are reabsorbed naturally, but as this happens new ones are formed. This kind of retinopathy does not affect vision. Vision is affected only when the blood vessel changes occur in the center of the retina.

Proliferative retinopathy is the more serious of the two forms. It affects only 3 to 10 percent of all diabetic people.

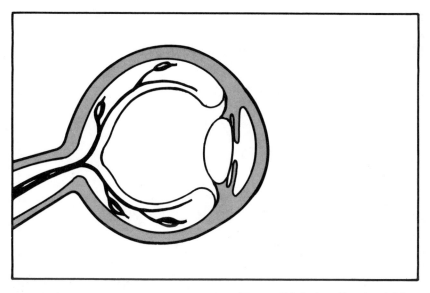

Figure 8–3. Background retinopathy. (From *Diabetes Forecast* 31 [6]: 1978)

The name describes the nature of the condition: New blood vessels grow by multiplication through the surface of the retina and sometimes protrude into the vitreous. These microaneurysms are fragile, and when they break, blood flows into the vitreous shutting off the light so that it cannot enter the eye. Although small hemorrhages are absorbed quickly when this occurs, some are never absorbed. New blood vessels grow in the vitreous at the sites of unabsorbed hemorrhages, and scar tissue builds in the vitreous and also in the retina. The weight and tension of the scar tissue can pull on the retina, causing it to draw away from the wall of the eye into the vitreous. Sight may not be lost if the new blood vessels are confined to the edges of the retina; however, if the retina becomes detached, then vision is lost (fig. 8–4).

Treatment for both types of retinopathy attempts to slow the growth of the new blood vessels by photocoagulation. The treatment depends upon the type of retinopathy, the general health of the patient, and the condition of other blood

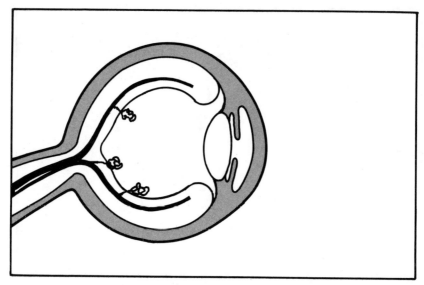

Figure 8–4. **Proliferative retinopathy. (Studies of the eye adapted from *Diabetes Forecast* 31 [6]: 1978)**

vessels in the body, particularly those affecting the heart and kidneys.

Photocoagulation is a scarring produced by intense laser light. The aim is to seal off the newly formed blood vessels. Photocoagulation has been found to be very helpful in slowing the growth of new blood vessels within the eye. It is not used, however, when the retina is covered with a cataract or in severe vitreous hemorrhage. Besides light treatment, there are effective medical treatments, such as better regulation of blood sugar, strict attention to diet, and prevention of infection, that are used in the treatment of retinopathy.

Vitrectomy is a surgical technique that is being used successfully to restore sight in those who have lost it due to vitreous hemorrhage and retinal detachment. Not everyone can be helped by this surgery, and patients must be carefully chosen to ensure a successful outcome.

The treatment of diabetic retinopathy has progressed greatly in the past 10 years, and studies are underway continuously to prevent loss of sight and to restore it whenever possible.

There is new hope for preventing diabetic retinopathy in a procedure currently under study by National Eye Institute investigators. In this procedure, circulation in the eye can be observed with the use of a dye injected into the bloodstream and measured by an electronic instrument called a fluorophotometer. When this technique is perfected and tested, it is hoped that early changes in the eye due to diabetes can be found and measures to prevent retinopathy can be taken.

Summary: While there is no proven way to positively prevent retinopathy, authorities agree that good diabetes control is an important factor in delaying the onset of eye disease. Diabetic patients should have regular (twice yearly) eye examinations by an ophthalmologist (a doctor who specializes in eye disorders) so that early retinal changes can be found and treatment started when necessary.

KIDNEY DISEASE

Diabetic nephropathy (disease of the kidneys) is a serious complication of diabetes. When it occurs it usually affects persons who have had diabetes for many years. Because the kidneys are capable of handling many times the normal amount of waste formed by the body, kidney disease can progress slowly and often without apparent symptoms.

The kidneys are small organs located on either side of the spine just above the waist. Their function is to filter waste products, chemicals, and water from the blood to form urine. Ureters, long slender tubes, carry the urine from the kidneys to the bladder, where it is stored until the urine is released from the body through the urethra. The kidneys, ureters, bladder, and urethra together form the urinary tract (fig. 8–5).

Each kidney is made up of glomeruli, tufts of tiny blood vessels which form the basis of the filtering system. Due to

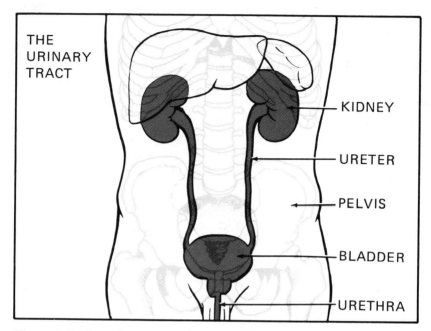

Figure 8-5. **The urinary tract. (From *Diabetes Forecast* 33 [3]: 1980)**

fluctuating blood sugar levels (in diabetes), the lining of the walls of these blood vessels sometimes changes over a period of time, causing the filtering capacity of the kidneys to decline. The blood vessels become thickened and porous, causing a loss of protein from the blood. This loss upsets the normal, delicate fluid balance in the body. As the kidneys lose more and more of their function, chemicals and wastes accumulate in the blood, which can harm tissue and cause lasting kidney damage. This condition is called glomerulosclerosis (hardening of the glomeruli) and only occurs in persons with diabetes. A doctor can often detect developing nephropathy by looking at the retina of the eye. Because diabetes affects the small blood vessels of both the retina of the eye and the kidney, any changes in the retina may indicate changes in the kidneys as well.

Other symptoms of nephropathy include pus cells, blood, casts and protein in the urine, swelling of the feet and ankles, persistent fatigue, a yellowish pallor of the skin, and often elevated blood pressure.

Another disorder of the kidneys that sometimes affects, but is not limited to, persons with diabetes is nephrosclerosis. This is a hardening of the arteries of the kidneys associated with high blood pressure and poorly functioning kidneys.

Some common urinary tract infections that are likely to affect diabetic people are pyelitis, an inflammation of the renal pelvis, the area where urine collects before it descends to the bladder; pyelonephritis, an inflammation of the glomeruli; and cystitis, an inflammation of the bladder. Diabetic people should be aware of the signs and symptoms of urinary tract infections: cloudy or bloody urine, an urgent need to urinate, painful urination, low pack pain, and fever. If these symptoms occur, a doctor should be called promptly. Early diagnosis of urinary tract infections, and prompt and thorough treatment, are essential to insure that no trace of infection remains that could cause the condition to become chronic.

What Is the Treatment for Kidney Disease?

Treatment consists of a careful review of total kidney function. The diet may be adjusted to help make up for the loss of protein and to assist the kidney's reduced capacity to remove waste products. Efforts are made to control high blood pressure, eliminate smoking, restrict salt in the diet, and maintain the best possible diabetes control to slow the progress of the disease.

If kidney failure does occur, the outlook is much brighter today than it was even a few years ago. Hemodialysis makes this possible. In this process the patient's blood is filtered and cleansed of all waste materials by an artificial kidney. In a controlled continuous flow, blood from the body is passed through the machine and returned to the body. This is a common practice today in the treatment of kidney failure. Hemodialysis treatments are usually carried out two or three times per week.

Kidney transplants have become fairly common in recent years and have proved very successful, particularly if a kidney from a living, related donor is used.

Is it possible to prevent kidney disease? There is hope now that diabetic kidney disease can be prevented. A recent study of a strain of mice subject to diabetes, obesity, and kidney disease, similar to the conditions found in humans with diabetes, showed that when obesity was prevented and blood glucose was closely controlled with diet, the diabetic changes in the kidney did not occur. Further research is needed, but the evidence is mounting that strict control in all aspects of diabetes may prevent many complications.

Summary: Kidney disease in diabetes is a serious complication. It is related to the duration of diabetes, the degree of control, and the presence of high blood pressure. While the decreased blood flow through the small blood vessels in the kidneys is not always caused by poor diabetes control, there is increasing proof that this is a factor. To avoid, minimize, or prevent permanent kidney damage, it is important for people with diabetes to be alert to the symptoms of developing kidney disease as well as those of urinary tract infection and to seek treatment promptly.

DISEASE OF THE NERVES: NEUROPATHY

Neuropathy is a common complication of diabetes which can affect many parts of the body. The term means physical disease of the nerves and has nothing to do with the emotions. Diabetic neuropathy appears to affect men more often than women. It is fairly uncommon among young people. The risk of developing it increases with the duration of diabetes. The symptoms are often severe and painful, but they tend to disappear in time when diabetes is brought under good control.

There are four types of neuropathy that can affect the nerves of the body: peripheral, autonomic, motor, and cranial. _Peripheral neuropathy_ is the most common type. It involves the outermost nerves of the body which connect the muscles, skin, blood vessels, and other organs to the spinal column. This type of neuropathy most often affects the legs and feet, and sometimes the hands. It is marked by numbness, tingling, weakness, and an intense pain described as similar to a toothache. The pain is usually more severe at night, causing a loss of sleep. It generally eases by morning, only to return again at nightfall. Pain and loss of sleep can be very depressing to the patient. When pain is severe the doctor may prescribe drugs for relief. These medications may also help to lift the depression associated with pain and sleep loss.

When peripheral neuropathy affects the feet, they can become so insensitive that pressure, pain, heat, and cold cannot be felt. For example, a stone inside the shoe can go unnoticed. When neuropathy affects the hands, it can cause a wasting of muscle tissue in the hand, making tasks such as typing, writing, or working with tools difficult.

When feeling is lost in the feet and toes, they can sometimes be injured, frozen, or burned, and the pain will not be felt. Hot water bottles and heating pads should not be used because they could cause serious burns. A blister or puncture wound on the foot can go unnoticed until it becomes infected. Neuropathic ulcers (open infected sores) can develop on the soles of the foot due to pressure spots or foreign objects inside the shoe. When feeling in the foot is lost, these ulcers can progress to a serious stage before they are noticed. It is very important for the patient with peripheral neuropathy to examine his/her feet daily. If skin breaks or ulcers do occur, a doctor or a podiatrist skilled in the treatment of foot problems should be seen immediately. Treatment usually consists of medication for the infection and corrective measures to relieve the pressure on the ulcer. To prevent ulcers, the feet should be kept clean, shoes should fit properly, and excess weight lost so as to lighten the burden of the feet.

Autonomic neuropathy involves the nerves that are not consciously controlled, such as those of the bladder, intestinal tract, and the genital organs. Paralysis of the bladder, caused by neuropathy, is a serious condition which needs prompt medical attention. One of the signs of this condition is repeated urinary tract infections. The nerves of the bladder lose the ability to respond normally to pressure as the bladder fills. The urine is retained in the bladder, causing bacterial infection, and if untreated, kidney damage results. Prompt treatment with drugs to overcome urine retention and antibiotics to treat the infection are used. Diabetic people should be alert to the symptoms of urinary tract infection and call their doctor promptly should symptoms appear (see section of kidney disease).

Diabetic diarrhea occurs when the nerves that control the small intestine are affected by neuropathy. The diarrhea occurs most often at night, and although it can be frequent and severe, it seldom upsets diabetes control, and it does not seem to have an ill effect on the general health. The course of this condition is irregular, getting better and worse from time to time before it finally goes away. Treatment consists of antidiarrhea drugs and antibiotics if needed.

Impotence, a complication of diabetes that may be caused by neuropathy, is more common in diabetic males past adolescence than in nondiabetic males. It should be stressed, however, that not all diabetic males become impotent, and all cases of impotence are not caused by diabetes.

Impotence is the inability to start, sustain, and complete the act of sexual intercourse. When the nerves controlling erection are affected by neuropathy, impotence often results. However, there are many causes for impotence, such as fear, anxiety, anger, injury, illness, hormonal deficiency, brain disease, drug reactions, and alcoholism. A doctor must determine the cause of the impotence before treatment can be started. If impotence is due to diabetes and the diabetes has been poorly controlled, the impotence may disappear once good control has been established. And, if the nerves have been damaged, there are surgical means that can restore function. After assessing the extent of the neuropathy, the doctor will be able to advise the patient on a course of treatment, including sexual and psychological counseling when needed.

Motor neuropathy affects the muscles, particularly of the thighs. When the nerves in these muscles are damaged the legs are weakened, and walking becomes difficult and painful. The symptoms include a burning sensation in the leg which may begin slowly or may appear suddenly. One or both legs may be affected. Recovery is slow and may take anywhere from 6 to 18 months. Although the pain is frequently severe, patients should know that it will eventually disappear. Treatment consists of drugs to relieve the pain and strict attention to good diabetes control. Strangely enough, although this type of neuropathy affects the legs, the arms are seldom involved.

Cranial neuropathy affects the nerves that control the eye muscles. The paralysis of these muscles may be preceded by pain in the side of the head near the affected eye. The double vision that occurs with the paralysis is caused by the eye muscles not working in unison. This is a very disturbing condition. The symptoms usually subside within 2 to 3 months, and recovery is usually complete. As in the other neuropathies, treatment consists of drugs to control the pain; when necessary, an eye patch is prescribed to make the condition more bearable.

Summary: Neuropathy is a general term for some serious and painful complications that occur in some people with diabetes. The causes are not clearly understood as yet; however, as in the other complications previously described, good control of diabetes is recommended to help delay and possibly prevent the onset of many of these problems.

9

DIABETES AND
THE FAMILY

Diabetes is an uninvited guest who comes to stay and can threaten everyone in the family. This unwelcome guest demands constant attention which can, in some circumstances, strain all the resources of the family. How the diabetic person and the family cope with this omnipresent guest has a profound effect on the outcome of the disease.

For many years research was focused on the effect of diabetes on the body. Increasingly, however, attention has been given to how it affects the spirit and the feelings, and how these feelings influence the physical course of the disease. It is now a firmly held belief that improved patient and family education, understanding of diabetes management and living with diabetes will lead to improved metabolic control, minimize short- and intermediate-term complications, and possibly reduce chronic complications.

PSYCHOSOCIAL ISSUES

How the person feels about his/her disease, how the family feels, and how they interact with each other and with the health professionals who care for them, are the crux of these issues. Feelings common to all newly diagnosed diabetic people are those of loss and grief that health has been taken away; fear and anxiety about the future; and feelings of helplessness, that "there is nothing I can do." Anger, denial, and guilt are not uncommon reactions to the diagnosis of diabetes, particularly on the part of parents who initially fail to realize that nothing they did caused their child's diabetes. The diabetic person who "cheats" on his/her prescribed diet may feel guilty when a high blood sugar appears but suffer anger and frustration if an emergency occurs when following all the rules. There are often feelings of resentment among siblings because the child with diabetes seems to get all the attention. Tension may arise between spouses because the diabetic person's physical care and needs always seem to come first. Fear of complications can haunt both diabetic people and their families.

RESOLVING CONFLICTS

The single most important factor in coping with both the physical and emotional impact of diabetes is *education*. Only when there is a clear understanding of what diabetes is, how it can be managed, how to prevent emergencies, and how to cope with complications should they arise, will these feelings begin to be resolved. The person with diabetes should learn as soon as possible to take full charge of his/her own care. In this task, encouragement and help from the health-care team and the family are necessary. This is particularly true in times of crisis, during emotional upsets due to fluctuating blood sugar, and in times of discouragement. Diabetes control can be affected adversely by both physical and emotional stress, and it is important that the family recognize, understand, and be ready to give loving support during stressful periods. The diabetic person, on the other hand, should not use diabetes to get attention or to disrupt the peace of the family, nor should he/she expect special consideration either in the family or outside because of diabetes.

The Madison Conference identified the following crisis times in the lives of persons with diabetes: the diagnosis, the start of school, adolescence, college and the first job, marriage, pregnancy, and the onset of complications. In each of these instances, the person with diabetes needs the loving, freely given support of family and friends and the expert help of a good health-care team.

COUNSELING

Parents of young diabetic children must assume responsibility for care until such time as the child can gradually take over injections, testing, and food selection. This happens when the individual child is ready. The experience of a summer camp for diabetic children is an excellent way for parents to help their diabetic child become independent.

Adolescents need particular love and understanding if diabetes is discovered during these years. The family has to act as a buffer, be firm, and yet make necessary allowances for the loss of emotional control which may be due to swings in blood sugar levels or to hormonal factors common to this period of rapid growth.

When serious difficulties arise with diabetic children and young people, counseling from someone outside the family often helps. A professional counselor, or perhaps another diabetic person who has experienced the same problems and has been able to overcome them successfully, will have an objective viewpoint. Parents should strive to make their diabetic child feel accepted. They should stress that while diabetes makes a physical difference, just as wearing glasses or a hearing aid might, it does not take away the human, loving qualities that make the child unique.

Rebellion during adolescence is not uncommon, and it takes a stable family to cope with it successfully. Young people want to be grown up, to be independent, but parents still hover and may be reluctant to let go. It can be a very trying time, but infinite patience, firmness, and a sense of humor will help. How many times parents are reproached with words like, "Why do you always have to know where I'm

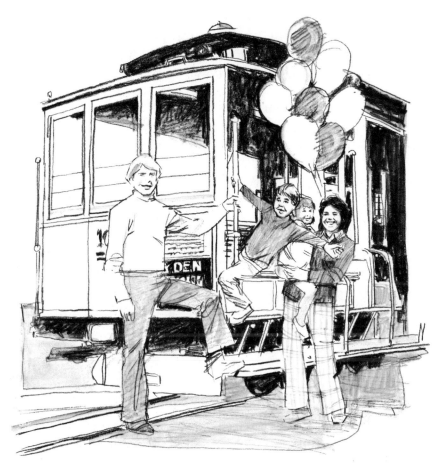

Figure 9–1. **An understanding happy family helps.**

going and when I'll be home? You just don't trust me." Time and trust are not the point, but as the parent, you can try to explain your feelings and concerns. You know your diabetic son is an excellent driver, but there are other less expert drivers on the road; your diabetic daughter is a superb skier, but this is the first ski weekend since her diabetes was discovered and you are not sure how strenuous exercise will affect her blood sugar control. Parents have feelings and are entitled to express them too.

Teenagers in particular suffer from a lack of self-esteem during these years, and diabetes frequently adds to their self-doubt. Parents need to reassure their teenagers often so confidence can be built. Group activities with other diabetic youth will help to show them that they are not facing diabetes alone. These activities also provide an opportunity for sports and a sharing of interests, both of which ease tensions.

When the young diabetic person enters the job market, he/she may experience discrimination, which can be a real setback to self-esteem. Whenever possible, young diabetic people should prepare for a career that is compatible with diabetes. Help in making a wise choice can be provided by the health-care team, the family, and the school counselor.

Marriage may be another crisis time in the life of the person with diabetes. It can either help or hurt the diabetes, depending upon the maturity of the partners. It is essential that the nondiabetic party have education in the management of diabetes and fully understand the responsibilities involved in living with a person who has diabetes.

While the diagnosis of diabetes in the middle years may not appear to be as devastating as in the adolescent years, it is a threat to the status quo. It is disconcerting to find that you have a chronic disease, particularly when you don't feel very ill. It is often difficult to change the habits of a lifetime with respect to eating, drinking, smoking, and physical exercise.

Diabetes in the elderly is frightening and bewildering because so often older people live alone. They may have no previous knowledge about diabetes or have preconceived or erroneous ideas, and learning may be difficult. The need to change the habits of a lifetime is often more than they can manage. Frequently, the diabetic diet and medications conflict with those prescribed for other health problems. Anxieties build because there is no one with whom they can talk. The elderly often suffer because of lack of knowledge of nutrition, or physical handicaps such as loss of teeth or poor dentures. The health-care team may have to be particularly careful to listen to and guide these people in the care and control of their diabetes. Whenever possible, a family member or close friend should be enlisted as a physical and moral support for the elderly person with diabetes.

Summary: Diabetes will always be an unwanted guest, but the family must learn to put this guest in the proper place and not permit diabetes to become the whole focus of the family.

In 1921 Randall Sprague developed diabetes at the age of 15. He says, "Every day of treatment in the preinsulin era involved either a starvation or semistarvation diet. In all I missed two years of school and was starved down to 78 pounds. It was a discouraging life for an adolescent boy, but I don't recall any tremendous psychological problems, possibly because I had the benefit of wise and loving parents and good medical care."

In 1922 he was one of the first diabetic people to receive insulin. Today, some 43,000 injections of insulin and 60 years later, Dr. Sprague enjoys emeritus status at the Mayo Clinic in Rochester, after a successful career in research and clinical medicine.

10

DIABETES IN LIFE STAGES

Living and surviving with diabetes is a continuous challenge, whether it is discovered early in life or late. From infancy to old age, life is an ongoing evolutionary process. Each year of growth imposes itself upon the last, building the human person much like a mason constructs a house by laying brick upon brick. New knowledge, changing physical skills and challenges, social development, crises, and problems that occur during a lifetime all contribute to the making of the individual as a person. No one would deny that living a full life with diabetes requires extra courage and stamina.

This chapter summarizes some of the most common characteristics in the life stages of the person with diabetes. Identifying with these various stages may provide you with some measure of objectivity and reassurance about your child's, another family member's, or your own diabetes.

DIABETES IN LIFE STAGES

Early Childhood

Social Characteristics
Parents should try to avoid overprotectiveness. Even at an early age the child can sense this.

Adjustment to diabetes is probably easiest for the child when diagnosed at this age.

Good eating habits, injections, and testing can become a normal part of the child's routine.

Physical Characteristics
Behavior: busy, active.
Food: intake erratic.

Growth: rapid; child is developing physically and socially.

Good eating habits should be established as early as possible.

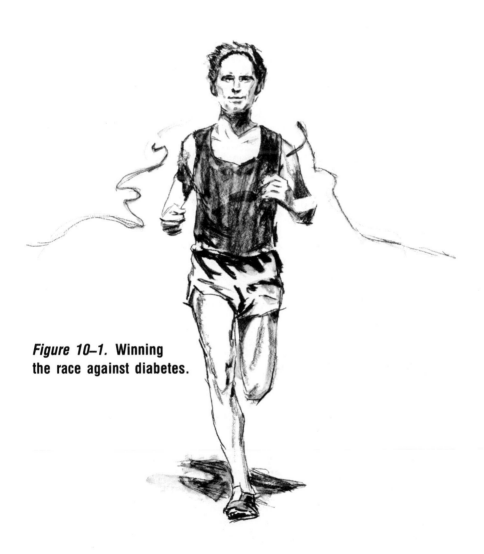

Figure 10–1. **Winning the race against diabetes.**

Special Considerations
Urine testing: difficult. Can use Tes-Tape® with cloth diaper. Both paper diapers that contain chemicals and cloth diapers washed in chlorine will give a false reading. Blood testing can be introduced gradually.

Difficult to understand child's response to symptoms. Is it hypo/hyperglycemia, or is the child just out of sorts?

Insulin reactions are more likely due to irregular eating and activity. A slight glucose spill is preferable to reactions at this time.

Elementary Years

Social Characteristics
Peer identification starts. Wanting to be just like others can cause problems with testing, injections, eating away from home, what to tell the teachers and friends about diabetes.

It is important for the child to be able to talk with others about diabetes. Child should be allowed "overnights" as soon as self-care is established.

Many children enjoy learning, and this helps in diabetes education for themselves and others.

Parents should avoid overprotectiveness now that the child is away from home more.

Children learn by example. Confidence, self-reliance, and performance are best achieved in an atmosphere of love, firmness, and good example.

Physical Characteristics
Activity pattern levels off.

Appetite is more constant.

Growth should be measured against standard charts.

Important to establish regular meals and snacks spaced throughout the day to meet the growing child's needs.

Special Considerations
Self-care can begin as soon as the child is ready. Testing, injections, and food selection (a choice at school cafeteria) should initially be done under the supervision of a parent. Attendance at summer camp will encourage independence.

Still some difficulty in understanding body feelings; for example, is the stomach ache due to diabetes or another physical problem, or a lack of enthusiasm for going to school?

With regular schedule of meals, snacks, and exercise, insulin reactions should be less likely. Child needs to carry some form of sugar when away from home for use in emergencies.

Parents need to meet with teachers to discuss the child's diabetes.

Adolescence

Social Characteristics
Anger and rebellion are common.

Acceptance of diabetes is most difficult for this age group.

Young persons should be encouraged to join ADA youth groups for peer support and better self-image.

Increasing independence. Young persons need to demonstrate ability to assume responsibilities. Parents need to provide backup support and the ability to listen.

A mature relationship between parents and children can be forged at this time, if parents stand by ready to give the occasional but necessary support, when asked.

Physical Characteristics
When teenage girls finish growing they need to reduce intake of insulin and calories in order to avoid a weight gain.

When girls, especially, deviate from the meal plan, it is preferable to go back to the plan rather than increase insulin.

Increased insulin only increases appetite, which leads to weight gain.

Calorie requirements for boys and girls vary greatly because of size and activity.

Appetite is the best guide to appropriate calorie levels.

Special Considerations
Rapid growth and hormonal changes may make diabetes more difficult to control.

Self-management of diabetes at this time can be a constructive part of "cutting the apron strings."

Avoid the use of alcohol, or use sparingly and with respect, always remembering to eat when drinking.

By taking full responsibility for diabetes, the young person demonstrates his/her ability to participate in sports, drive a car, and enjoy increased independence.

Sex education and avoidance of early pregnancy are important.

Young Adulthood

Social Characteristics
Marriage and genetic counseling will help in coping with problems of diabetes and possibility of children developing diabetes.

Discrimination and unemployment can occur. Job retraining and skill development possible through government agencies. Important to know how to handle these situations. The local ADA affiliate can help.

Life and health insurance are important.

Securing coverage may be difficult because of diabetes. Group plans are easiest to get into. Most employers provide group plans today.

Physical Characteristics
When growth is complete, diabetes becomes easier to control.

Maintenance of desirable body weight is essential because insulin is used more effectively.

Physical activity is usually reduced when school days are over, but some form of regular exercise should be established and adhered to.

Special Considerations
Getting established in a job or career makes emotional and physical demands that can affect diabetes.

Good diabetes control is essential in handling new challenges and responsibilities.

Marriage makes special demands. Both partners must understand diabetes and be willing to accept the added responsibilities that it requires.

Pregnancy creates special needs: added nutritional requirements, medical supervision, and added expense. Plan ahead for physical, emotional, and financial demands.

Middle Age

Social Characteristics
Coping with losses difficult.

Loss of health/diabetes.

Children leaving home.

Death of parents.

Possible death of a spouse.

Changes in life-style due to diabetes viewed as loss.

Loss of status, competition with younger people on the job.

Need to improve the quality of life: learn enjoyment of little things; find ways to relax tensions—hobby or relaxation techniques.

Physical Characteristics
Diabetes difficult to accept. It interrupts the established flow of life.

Obesity is often a problem. Changing eating, drinking, smoking, and exercise habits of a lifetime difficult. Often little motivation to do so because the person does not feel ill.

Special Considerations
Impotence may occur at this time. May be due to diabetes or other factors.

Menopause may require changes in diabetes medication.

Good foot care is essential. Serious problems are more likely to arise at this time.

Elderly

Social Characteristics
Family support is essential. If the elderly person lives alone, provision should be made for a relative or friend to make regular visits.

Depression common in the elderly. Need to ward off by encouraging activity, intellectual and physical, according to ability. Participation in community and senior citizen activities important.

Lifetime hobbies help now.

Quality of life very important.

Health-care providers need to be patient and generous with their time and help.

Physical Characteristics
Diabetes discovered now is frightening. In many cases it is just one more sickness added to other ills that already beset the person.

Proper nutrition is very important but frequently hard to achieve. Lack of knowledge, conflicting dietary restrictions for concomitant health problems cause confusion. Faulty dentures and reduced income only add to the problem.

Special Considerations
Drug reactions possible, particularly where there are concomitant physical problems.

Blood vessel disease, foot problems, high blood pressure, impotence, and eye problems are all causes of grave concern.

Treatment should aim to relieve diabetes symptoms with reasonable but not overly strict emphasis on blood sugar control.

11

THE PROMISE
OF RESEARCH

People with diabetes are living longer and healthier lives today, thanks to diabetes research. In particular:

- Women with diabetes are having more and healthier babies.
- Laser therapy is saving the eyesight of countless individuals with diabetic retinopathy.
- Self-monitoring of blood glucose is helping individuals prevent hypoglycemia and hyperglycemia.
- Insulins have been purified and even genetically engineered.
- Portable insulin pumps that deliver slow steady doses of insulin and short bursts on computer instruction are helping wearers mimic "normal" insulin delivery, and thereby improve control.

The list is endless, and the research that led to these and other life-enhancing discoveries is continuing.

What follows are highlights of areas in which exciting research is currently being conducted.

GENETICS AND IMMUNOLOGY

From previous research, we now know that insulin-dependent (Type I) diabetes is an autoimmune disease that strikes individuals with a certain genetic makeup. This means that simply having certain genes makes a person susceptible to developing diabetes. Researchers are seeking to identify the precise genes responsible for insulin-dependent diabetes and to determine what mechanisms trigger an individual's immune system to mistakenly destroy the beta cells (insulin-producing cells) of the pancreas.

Immunology researchers are trying to determine how to stop the destruction of beta cells before it is complete. One way you may have heard about is *immunosuppression,* an experimental therapy in which individuals whose diabetes is newly diagnosed are given powerful drugs that prevent the immune system from working. Generally, these people have some remaining beta cells. Stopping the immune system at this point keeps the remaining beta cells intact, and thus reduces or even eliminates the need for insulin. This treatment appears to work in individuals whose insulin-dependent diabetes has just been diagnosed—as long as the individuals keep taking the drugs. However, suppressing the immune system leaves these individuals open to nausea, infections, abnormalities of white blood cell production, an increased risk of cancer, and other harmful side effects.

In addition, immunosuppression is a prevention, not a cure. This means that even if this therapy were to become viable, it would only prevent new cases of diabetes; it cannot rejuvenate beta cells that have been destroyed. The cure for people who already have diabetes will have to come from another arena.

TRANSPLANTS

Transplantation is becoming a commonplace therapy in the treatment of many diseases, and diabetes is no exception. At present, two different types of transplants are under study and the future looks bright. But both pancreas and islet cell transplants are still experimental and much more study is necessary before this treatment becomes standard.

Pancreas transplants appear the most successful to date. Studies show long-term (1 year or more) survival rates of the transplanted organ are quite good and continue to get better. The greatest obstacle to success with transplants is rejection. The body tries to reject the transplanted organ it sees as foreign; it also may repeat the mistake that leads to diabetes and destroy the beta cells of the transplanted pancreas. Transplant researchers are looking to the immunology experts for answers. They also are looking at more effective ways of matching donor organs to recipients.

The other approach involves transplanting groups of individual islet cells rather than the pancreas. These islet cells can be rejected, just like the pancreas. But scientists are trying to prevent rejection by sealing the cells in porous capsules. The pores are big enough to let insulin and glucose pass through, but small enough to keep out cells that cause rejection. Despite some promising results in animal tests, capsules tend to become coated with cells that stop the release of insulin. Researchers are now trying to find a material for making capsules that will be more compatible with the body.

IMPLANTABLE GLUCOSE SENSOR/PUMP

A device about the size of a quarter may someday make life much simpler for people with insulin-dependent diabetes. Work on an implantable artificial beta cell/glucose sensor, a mechanical device that imitates the natural function of the pancreas, has been underway for more than a decade now. The device is so complicated that its development has required the expertise of electrochemists, chemical engineers, pathologists, physiologists, and clinical investigators. When perfected, this tiny device will include a reservoir to hold insulin, a pump for the delivery of insulin, and a sensor to monitor blood glucose levels and release the right amount of insulin in response to the body's needs. The mechanical portion of the device has been perfected. Now, researchers are seeking a porous membrane such as the one needed to encase transplanted islet cells.

In the meantime, scientists are working on a programmable, implantable medication system (called PIMS). This computerized device could free people from the need to carry an external insulin pump. PIMS looks like a hockey puck, about 3 inches in diameter and less than 1 inch thick. It is surgically implanted in the abdomen, and holds enough insulin so that refills are necessary only 4 to 5 times per year. The doctor or person with diabetes uses a radio transmitter to adjust the insulin flow. This device is not a glucose sensor, and a person using it must still do self-monitoring of blood glucose. The device is still being tested.

NUTRITION

Because diabetes affects the way food is processed, nutrition experts are studying how the body breaks down and uses food. This area of study has already led to some changes in the way we think about food and its effect on diabetes control. A prime example is the 1986 updating of the Exchange Lists for Meal Planning. New analyses have allowed food scientists to more thoroughly evaluate the nutrient content in specific foods to make the lists more accurate.

Another key topic is fiber. Nutritional scientisits are now investigating the benefits of fiber, the part of food not digested in the intestine. Some studies have shown that fiber, especially soluble fiber found in fruits, beans, and oat products, can help control blood glucose levels. It may also reduce requirements for insulin and other medication. Other studies suggest that following a high-fiber diet may help reduce blood cholesterol levels. However, not all research groups investigating fiber have found positive effects. And fiber is not recommended for certain people. For example, people with diabetic neuropathy (nerve damage) should check with their doctor before adding fiber to the diet. Scientists are stepping up efforts to learn more about fiber in relation to diabetes.

A tool to help your dietitian create individualized meal plans is still in development, but you've probably heard about it. The glycemic index is a scale for measuring the power of different foods to raise blood glucose levels. When it was introduced, some researchers argued that the glycemic index might be a better tool for meal planning than the Exchange Lists. They pointed to studies showing that foods within each exchange list can affect blood glucose levels very differently. Not all studies have shown the effectiveness of the glycemic index, however. Until all the data are in, the glycemic index remains primarily a tool for researchers.

INSULIN RESISTANCE

Many people with non-insulin-dependent (Type II) diabetes face the problem of having too much insulin because their bodies don't recognize insulin or their insulin receptors have closed down. What causes the body to lock insulin out is still a mystery, but researchers are studying the process of molecular binding (how one cell attaches itself to another) and what happens afterward in the cell.

OBESITY

The link between obesity (being more than 20 percent over ideal body weight) and developing diabetes in people who are genetically susceptible is undeniable. But what is it about obesity that prompts diabetes? Current research is underway to examine all aspects of this relationship, from the nervous system to the function of fat cells.

When and where the next research advance will come from is anybody's guess. That's why the American Diabetes Association supports researchers around the country in a variety of fields. The ADA is the leading voluntary health agency supporting diabetes research in this country. Along with funding research directly, the Asssociation uses its network of affiliates, chapters, and its National Service Center to keep open lines of communications with lawmakers to ensure necessary funds for the National Institutes of Health and other federal agencies involved in diabetes-related research and care.

12 RESOURCES

A BASIC MEAL PLAN

It is important to understand that you don't have to prepare special meals just because there is a person with diabetes in the family. A good, basic, nutritional meal plan can be adapted to meet the needs of the entire family. Following is an example of a one-day plan for an imaginary family that includes a diabetic father, a slightly overweight mother, an active, athletic teenage son, and a lively and energetic pre-teen daughter.

Breakfast	Lunch	Dinner
Orange juice or raisins	Hamburger	Chicken Cacciatore,*
Raisin or whole wheat	Sesame seed bun	tomatoes, and celery
bread	Vegetable plate: sliced	Potato
Margarine	tomatoes, onions,	Green beans
Jelly	carrot sticks, and	Cornbread muffin
Hot oatmeal	cauliflower bits	Margarine
Sugar	Margarine	Jelly
Skim milk	Mustard	Pear halves
Pecans	Apple	Pound cake
	Graham crackers	
	Skim milk	

*Recipe from *ADA Family Cookbook* (New York: Prentice Hall Press, 1986), 123.

The diabetic father (Type II) on a 1,500 calorie meal plan made up of 50 percent carbohydrate, 35 percent fat, and 15 percent protein, would select the following from the day's basic meal plan.

Meal	Carbohydrate	Protein	Fat	Calories	Total
Breakfast					
½ cup orange juice or 2 tbsp. raisins	15	—	—	60	
2 slices whole wheat toast	30	6	—	160	
2 tsp. margarine	—	—	10	90	
½ cup hot oatmeal	15	3	—	80	
1 cup skim milk	12	8	—	90	480
Lunch					
2-oz. hamburger patty	—	14	10	150	
1 small sesame seed bun	30	6	—	160	
Vegetable platter: sliced tomato, onion, carrot sticks, cauliflorettes	5	2	—	25	
1 tsp. margarine				45	
Mustard	free				
1 apple	15	—	—	60	
Coffee, tea, or Lo-cal drink					440
Dinner					
3 oz. chicken cacciatore (chicken breast, no skin, tomatoes, and celery)	12	24	9	245	
1 potato	15	3	—	80	
½ cup green beans	5	2	—	25	
1 cornbread muffin	15	3	—	80	
2 tsp. margarine	—	—	10	90	
2 pear halves	15	—	—	60	580
		Total daily cals.			1,500

Exchanges	Milk	Fruit	Vegetables	Starch/Bread	Meat	Fat
Breakfast	1	1		3		
Lunch	1	1	1	2	2M	1
Dinner		1	2	3½	3L	2

How the Rest of the Imaginary Family Might Eat

The mother who is watching her weight might take the same portions as her diabetic husband but omit either the oatmeal or toast at breakfast, and of course skip both the sugar and the jelly. At lunch she might take only a half of the sesame seed bun and omit the graham crackers and milk. At dinner she would choose either the potato or the muffin and omit the pound cake.

The son and daughter would probably eat everything in the day's plan, with the son taking slightly larger portions than his father and maybe even coming back for "seconds."

EXCHANGE LISTS FOR MEAL PLANNING

Starch/Bread List

Each item in this list contains about 15 grams of carbohydrate, 3 grams of protein, a trace of fat, and 80 calories. Whole grain products average about 2 grams of fiber per serving. Some foods are higher in fiber.

You can choose your starch servings from any of the items on this list. If you want to eat a starch food that is not on this list, the general rule is that:

- ½ cup of cereal, grain, or pasta is one serving.
- 1 ounce of a bread product is one serving.

Your dietitian can help you be more exact.

Cereals/Grains/Pasta

Bran cereals,* concentrated (such as Bran Buds®, All Bran®)	⅓ cup
Bran cereals,* flaked	½ cup
Bulgur (cooked)	½ cup
Cooked cereals	½ cup
Cornmeal (dry)	2½ tbsp.
Grapenuts®	3 tbsp.
Grits (cooked)	½ cup
Other ready-to-eat unsweetened cereals	¾ cup
Pasta (cooked)	½ cup
Puffed cereal	1½ cup
Rice, white or brown (cooked)	⅓ cup
Shredded wheat	½ cup
Wheat germ*	3 tbsp.

*3 grams or more of fiber per serving.

Dried Beans/Peas/Lentils

Beans* and peas* (cooked), such as white, split, blackeye, kidney	⅓ cup
Lentils* (cooked)	⅓ cup
Baked beans*	¼ cup

Starchy Vegetables

Corn*	½ cup
Corn on cob,* 6 in. long	1
Lima beans*	½ cup
Peas, green* (canned or frozen)	½ cup
Plantain*	½ cup
Potato, baked	1 small (3 oz.)
Potato, mashed	½ cup
Squash, winter* (acorn, butternut)	¾ cup
Yam, sweet potato, plain	⅓ cup

Bread

Bagel	½ (1 oz.)
Bread sticks, crisp, 4 in. long × ½ in. wide	2 (⅔ oz.)
Croutons, lowfat	1 cup
English muffin	½
Frankfurter or hamburger bun	½ (1 oz.)
Pita, 6 in. across	½
Plain roll, small	1 (1 oz.)
Raisin, unfrosted	1 slice (1 oz.)
Rye,* pumpernickel*	1 slice (1 oz.)
Tortilla, 6 in. across	1
White (including French, Italian)	1 slice (1 oz.)
Whole wheat	1 slice (1 oz.)

Crackers/Snacks

Animal crackers	8
Graham crackers, 2½-in. square	3
Matzoth	¾ oz.
Melba toast	5 slices
Oyster crackers	24
Popcorn (popped, no fat added)	3 cups
Pretzels	¾ oz.
Rye crisp, 2 in. × 3½ in.	4
Saltine-type crackers	6
Whole wheat crackers, no fat added (crisp breads, such as Finn®, Kavli®, Wasa®)	2–4 slices (¾ oz.)

*3 grams or more of fiber per serving.

Starch Foods Prepared with Fat
(Count as 1 starch/bread serving, plus 1 fat serving.)

Biscuit, 2½ in. across	1
Chow mein noodles	½ cup
Corn bread, 2-in. cube	1 (2 oz.)
Cracker, round butter type	6
French fried potatoes, 2 in. to 3½ in. long	10 (1½ oz.)
Muffin, plain, small	1
Pancake, 4 in. across	2
Stuffing, bread (prepared)	¼ cup
Taco shell, 6 in. across	2
Waffle, 4½-in. square	1
Whole wheat crackers, fat added (such as Triscuits®)	4–6 (1 oz.)

Meat List

Each serving of meat and substitutes on this list contains about 7 grams of protein. The amount of fat and number of calories varies, depending on what kind of meat or substitute you use. The list is divided into three parts, based on the amount of fat and calories: lean meat, medium-fat meat, and high-fat meat. One ounce (one meat exchange) of each of these includes:

	Carbohydrate (grams)	Protein (grams)	Fat (grams)	Calories
Lean	0	7	3	55
Medium-Fat	0	7	5	75
High-Fat	0	7	8	100

You are encouraged to use more lean and medium-fat meat, poultry, and fish in your meal plan. This will help decrease your fat intake, which may help decrease your risk for heart disease. The items from the high-fat group are high in saturated fat, cholesterol, and calories. You should limit your choices from the high-fat group to three (3) times per week. Meat and substitutes do not contribute any fiber to your meal plan.

Tips

- Bake, roast, broil, grill, or boil these foods rather than frying them with added fat.
- Use a nonstick pan spray or a nonstick pan to brown or fry these foods.
- Trim off visible fat before and after cooking.
- Do not add flour, bread crumbs, coating mixes, or fat to these foods when preparing them.
- Weigh meat after removing bones and fat, and after cooking. Three ounces of cooked meat is equal to about 4 ounces of raw meat. Some examples of meat portions are:

2 oz. meat (2 meat = 1 small chicken leg or thigh
    exchanges   ½ cup cottage cheese or tuna
3 oz. meat (3 meat = 1 medium pork chop
    exchanges   1 small hamburger
    ½ chicken breast (1 side)
    1 unbreaded fish fillet, cooked meat about the size of a deck of cards

- Restaurants usually serve prime cuts of meat, which are high in fat and calories.

Lean Meat and Substitutes
(One exchange is equal to any one of the following items.)

Beef	USDA good or choice grades of lean beef, such as round, sirlion, flank steak, tenderloin, chipped beef.*	1 oz.
Pork	Lean pork, such as fresh ham, canned, cured, or boiled ham,* Canadian bacon,* tenderloin.	1 oz.
Veal	All cuts are lean except for veal cutlets (ground or cubed). Examples of lean veal are chops and roasts.	1 oz.
Poultry	Chicken, turkey, Cornish hen (without skin)	1 oz.

*400 milligrams or more of sodium per exchange.

Fish	All fresh and frozen fish	1 oz.
	Crab, lobster, scallops, shrimp, clams (fresh, or canned in water*)	2 oz.
	Oysters	6 medium
	Tuna* (canned in water)	¼ cup
	Herring (uncreamed or smoked)	1 oz.
	Sardines (canned)	2 medium
Wild Game	Venison, rabbit, squirrel	1 oz.
	Pheasant, duck, goose (without skin)	1 oz.
Cheese	Any cottage cheese	¼ cup
	Grated parmesan	2 tbsp.
	Diet cheeses* with less than 55 calories per ounce	1 oz.
Other	95% fat-free luncheon meat*	1 oz.
	Egg whites	3 whites
	Egg substitutes with less than 55 calories per ¼ cup	¼ cup

Medium-Fat Meat and Substitutes
(One exchange is equal to any one of the following items.)

Beef	Most beef products fall into this category. Examples are: all gound beef, roast (rib, chuck, rump), steak (cubed, Porterhouse, T-bone), and meatloaf	1 oz.
Pork	Most pork products fall into this category. Examples are: chops, loin roast, Boston butt, cutlets	1 oz.
Lamb	Most lamb products fall into this category. Examples are: chops, leg, and roast.	1 oz.
Veal	Cutlet (ground or cubed, unbreaded)	1 oz.
Poultry	Chicken (with skin), domestic duck, or good (well-drained of fat) ground turkey	1 oz.
Fish	Tuna* (canned in oil and drained), salmon* (canned)	¼ cup
Cheese	Skim or part-skim milk cheeses, such as:	
	Ricotta	¼ cup
	Mozzarella	1 oz.
	Diet cheeses* with 56 to 80 calories per ounce	1 oz.

*400 milligrams or more of sodium per exchange.

Other	86 percent fat-free luncheon meat*	1 oz.
	Egg (high in cholesterol, limit to 3 per week)	1
	Egg substitutes with 56 to 80 calories per ¼ cup	¼ cup
	Tofu (2½ in. × 2¾ in. × 1 in.)	4 oz.
	Liver, heart, kidney, sweetbreads (high in cholesterol)	1 oz.

High-Fat Meat and Substitutes
Remember, these items are high in saturated fat, cholesterol, and calories and should be used only three (3) times per week. (One exchange is equal to any one of the following items.)

Beef	Most USDA prime cuts of beef, such as ribs, corned beef*	1 oz.
Pork	Spareribs, ground pork, pork sausage* (patty or link)	1 oz.
Lamb	Patties (ground lamb)	1 oz.
Fish	Any dried fish product	1 oz.
Cheese	All regular cheeses,* such as American, Blue, Cheddar, Monterey, Swiss	1 oz.
Other	Luncheon meat,* such as bologna, salami, pimento loaf	1 oz.
	Sausage,* such as Polish, Italian, smoked	1 oz.
	Knockwurst, smoked	1 oz.
	Bratwurst*	1 oz.
	Frankfurter* (turkey or chicken)	1 frank (10/lb)
	Peanut butter (contains unsaturated fat)	1 tablespoon

Count as one high-fat meat plus one fat exchange:

| | Frankfurter* (beef, pork, or combination) | 1 frank (10/lb.) |

Vegetable List

Each vegetable serving on this list contains about 5 grams of carbohydrate, 2 grams of protein, 25 calories, and 2 to 3 grams of dietary fiber.

Vegetables are a good source of vitamins and minerals. Fresh and frozen vegetables have more vitamins and less

*400 milligrams or more of sodium per serving.

added salt than canned vegetables. Rinsing canned vegetables will remove much of the salt.

Unless otherwise noted, the serving size for vegetables is:

- ½ cup of cooked vegetables or vegetable juice
- 1 cup of raw vegetables

Artichoke (½ medium)	Mushrooms, cooked
Asparagus	Okra
Beans (green, wax, Italian)	Onions
Bean sprouts	Pea pods
Beets	Peppers (green)
Broccoli	Rutabaga
Brussels sprouts	Sauerkraut*
Cabbage, cooked	Spinach, cooked
Carrots	Summer squash (crookneck)
Cauliflower	Tomato (one large)
Eggplant	Tomato/vegetable juice*
Greens (collard, mustard, turnip)	Turnip
Kohlrabi	Water chestnuts
Leeks	Zucchini, cooked

Starchy vegetables such as corn, peas, and potatoes are found on the Starch/Bread list.

For free vegetables, see Free Food list on page 170.

Fruit List

Each item on this list contains about 15 grams of carbohydrate and 60 calories. Fresh, frozen, and dried fruits have about 2 grams of fiber per serving. Fruit juices contain very little dietary fiber.

The carbohydrate and calorie contents for a fruit serving are based on the usual serving of the most commonly eaten fruits. Use fresh fruits or fruits frozen or canned without sugar added. Whole fruit is more filling than fruit juice and may be a better choice for those who are trying to lose weight. Unless otherwise noted, the serving size for fruit is:

- ½ cup of fresh fruit or fruit juice
- ¼ cup of dried fruit

*400 milligrams or more of sodium per serving.

Fresh, frozen, and unsweetened canned fruit

Apple (raw, 2 in. across)	1
Applesauce (unsweetened)	½ cup
Apricots (medium, raw)	4
Apricots (canned)	½ cup or 4 halves
Banana (9 in. long)	½
Blackberries* (raw)	¾ cup
Blueberries* (raw)	¾ cup
Cantaloupe (5 in. across)	⅓
(cubes)	1 cup
Cherries (large, raw)	12
Cherries (canned)	½ cup
Figs (raw, 2 in. across)	2
Fruit cocktail (canned)	½ cup
Grapefruit (medium)	½
Grapefruit (segments)	¾ cup
Grapes (small)	15
Honeydew melon (medium)	⅛ melon
(cubes)	1 cup
Kiwi (large)	1
Mandarin oranges	¾ cup
Mango (small)	½
Nectarine* (1½ in. across)	1
Orange (2½ in. across)	1
Papaya	1 cup
Peach (2¾ in. across)	1 peach, or ¾ cup
Peaches (canned)	½ cup, or 2 halves
Pear	½ large, or 1 small
Pears (canned)	½ cup, or 2 halves
Persimmon (medium, native)	2
Pineapple (raw)	¾ cup
Pineapple (canned)	⅓ cup
Plum (raw, 2 inches across)	2
Pomegranate*	½
Raspberries* (raw)	1 cup
Strawberries* (raw, whole)	1¼ cup
Tangerine* (2½ in. across)	2
Watermelon (cubes)	1¼ cup

Dried Fruit

Apples*	4 rings
Apricots*	7 halves
Dates	2½ medium
Figs*	1½
Prunes*	3 medium
Raisins	2 tbsp.

*3 grams or more of fiber per serving.

Fruit Juice

Apple juice/cider	½ cup
Cranberry juice cocktail	⅓ cup
Grapefruit juice	½ cup
Grape juice	⅓ cup
Orange juice	½ cup
Pineapple juice	½ cup
Prune juice	⅓ cup

Milk List

Each serving of milk or milk products on this list contains about 12 grams of carbohydrate and 8 grams of protein. The amount of fat in milk is measured in percent of butterfat. The calories vary, depending on what kind of milk you choose. The list is divided into three parts, based on the amount of fat and calories: skim/very lowfat milk, lowfat milk, and whole milk. One serving (one milk exchange) of each of these includes:

	Carbohydrate (grams)	Protein (grams)	Fat (grams)	Calories
Skim/Very Lowfat	12	8	trace	90
Lowfat	12	8	5	120
Whole	12	8	8	150

Milk is the body's main source of calcium, the mineral needed for growth and repair of bones. Yogurt is also a good source of calcium. Yogurt and many dry or powdered milk products have different amounts of fat. If you have questions about a particular item, read the label to find out the fat and calorie content.

Milk is good to drink, but it can also be added to cereal and to other foods. Many tasty dishes such as sugar-free pudding are made with milk. Plain yogurt is delicious with one of your fruit servings mixed with it.

Skim and Very Lowfat Milk

Skim milk	1 cup
½% milk	1 cup
1% milk	1 cup
Lowfat buttermilk	1 cup
Evaporated skim milk	½ cup
Dry nonfat milk	⅓ cup
Plain nonfat yogurt	8 oz.

Lowfat Milk

2% milk	1 cup
Plain lowfat yogurt	8 oz.
(with added nonfat milk solids)	

Whole Milk

The whole milk group has much more fat per serving than the skim and lowfat groups. Whole milk has more than 3¼ percent butterfat. Try to limit your choices from the whole milk group as much as possible.

Whole milk	1 cup
Evaporated whole milk	½ cup
Whole plain yogurt	8 oz.

Fat List

Each serving on the fat list contains about 5 grams of fat and 45 calories.

The foods on the fat list contain mostly fat, although some items may also contain a small amount of protein. All fats are high in calories and should be carefully measured. Everyone should modify fat intake by eating unsaturated fats instead of saturated fats. The sodium content of these foods varies widely. Check the label for sodium information.

Unsaturated Fats

Avocado	⅛ medium
Margarine	1 tsp.
Margarine, diet*	1 tbsp.
Mayonnaise	1 tsp.
Mayonnaise, reduced-calorie*	1 tbsp.
Nuts and Seeds	
Almonds, dry-roasted	6 whole
Cashews, dry-roasted	1 tbsp.
Pecans	2 whole
Peanuts	20 small, 10 large
Walnuts	2 whole
Other nuts	1 tbsp.
Seeds, pine nuts, sunflower (without shells)	1 tbsp.
Pumpkin seeds	2 tsp.
Oil (corn, cottonseed, safflower, soybean, sunflower, olive, peanut)	1 tsp.
Olives*	10 small, 5 large
Salad dressing, mayonnaise-type	2 tsp.
Salad dressing, mayonnaise-type, reduced-calorie	1 tbsp.
Salad dressing (all varieties)*	1 tbsp.
Salad dressing, reduced-calorie**	2 tbsp.

(Two tablespoons of low-calorie salad dressing is a free food.)

Saturated Fats

Butter	1 tsp.
Bacon*	1 slice
Chitterlings	½ oz.
Coconut, shredded	2 tbsp.
Coffee whitener, liquid	2 tbsp.
Coffee whitener, powder	4 tsp.
Cream (light)	2 tbsp.
Cream, sour	2 tbsp.
Cream (heavy, whipping)	1 tbsp.
Cream cheese	1 tbsp.
Salt pork*	¼ oz.

   *If more than one or two servings are consumed, sodium levels will equal or exceed 400 milligrams.
   **400 milligrams or more of sodium per serving.

Free Foods

A free food is any food or drink that contains 20 calories or less per serving. You may eat as much as you want of those items that have no serving size specified. You may eat two or three servings per day of those items that have a specific serving size. Be sure to spread them out through the day.

Drinks

Bouillon,* or broth without fat
Bouillon, low-sodium
Carbonated drinks, sugar-free
Carbonated water
Club soda
Cocoa powder, unsweetened (1 tbsp.)
Coffee/Tea
Drink mixes, sugar-free
Mineral water
Tonic water, sugar-free

Nonstick pan spray

Fruit

Cranberries, unsweetened (½ cup)
Rhubarb, unsweetened (½ cup)

Sweet Substitutes

Candy, hard, sugar-free
Gelatin, sugar-free
Gum, sugar-free
Jam/Jelly, sugar-free (2 tsp.)
Pancake syrup, sugar-free (1 to 2 tbsp.)
Sugar substitutes (saccharin, aspartame)
Whipped topping, low-calorie (2 tbsp.)

Vegetables (raw, 1 cup)

Cabbage
Celery
Chinese cabbage**
Cucumber
Green onion
Hot peppers
Mushrooms
Radishes
Zucchini**
Salad greens
  Endive
  Escarole
  Lettuce
  Romaine
  Spinach

Condiments

Catsup (1 tbsp.)
Horseradish
Mustard
Pickles,* dill, unsweetened
Salad dressing, low-calorie (2 tbsp.)
Taco sauce (1 tbsp.)
Vinegar

*400 milligrams or more of sodium per serving.
**3 grams or more of fiber per serving.

Seasonings can be very helpful in making food taste better. Be careful of how much sodium you use. Read the label, and choose those seasonings that do not contain sodium or salt.

Basil (fresh)
Celery seeds
Cinnamon
Chili powder
Chives
Curry
Dill
Flavoring extracts (vanilla, lemon, almond, walnut, peppermint, butter, and the like)
Garlic
Garlic powder
Herbs
Hot pepper sauce
Lemon
Lemon juice
Lemon pepper
Lime
Lime juice
Mint
Onion powder
Oregano
Paprika
Pepper
Pimento
Spices
Soy sauce*
Soy sauce, low-sodium
Wine, used in cooking (¼ cup)
Worcestershire sauce

Combination Foods

Much of the food we eat is mixed together in various combinations. These combination foods do not fit into only one Exchange List. It can be quite hard to tell what is in a certain casserole dish or baked food item. This is a list of average values for some typical combination foods. This list will help you fit these foods into your meal plan. Ask your dietitian for information about any other foods you would like to eat. The *American Diabetes Association/American Dietetic Association Family Cookbooks* and the *American Diabetes Association Holiday Cookbook* have numerous recipes and further information about many foods, including combination foods. Check your library or local bookstore.

*400 milligrams or more of sodium per serving.

Food	Amount	Exchanges
Casseroles, homemade	1 cup (8 oz.)	2 starch, 2 medium-fat meat, 1 fat
Cheese pizza,** thin crust	¼ of 15 oz. or ¼ of 10 in.	2 starch, 1 medium-fat meat, 1 fat
Chili with beans* ** (commercial)	1 cup (8 oz.)	2 starch, 2 medium-fat meat, 2 fat
Chow mein* ** (without noodles or rice)	2 cups (16 oz.)	1 starch, 2 vegetable, 2 lean meat
Macaroni and cheese**	1 cup (8 oz.)	2 starch, 1 medium-fat meat, 2 fat
Soup		
Bean* **	1 cup (8 oz.)	1 starch, 1 vegetable, 1 lean meat
Chunky, all varieties**	10¾ oz. can	1 starch, 1 vegetable, 1 medium-fat meat
Cream** (made with water)	1 cup (8 oz.)	1 starch, 1 fat
Vegetable ** or broth type**	1 cup (8 oz.)	1 starch
Spaghetti and meatballs (canned)	1 cup (8 oz.)	2 starch, 1 medium-fat meat, 1 fat
Sugar-free pudding (made with skim milk)	½ cup	1 starch
If beans are used as a meat substitute:		
Dried beans,* peas,* lentils*	1 cup (cooked)	2 starch, 1 lean meat

* 3 grams or more of fiber per serving.
** 400 milligrams or more of sodium per serving.

Foods for Occasional Use

Moderate amounts of some foods can be used in your meal plan, in spite of their sugar or fat content, as long as you can maintain blood-glucose control. The following list includes average exchange values for some of these foods. Because they are concentrated sources of carbohydrate, you will notice that the portion sizes are very small. Check with your dietitian for advice on how often and when you can eat them.

Food	Amount	Exchanges
Angel food cake	¹⁄₁₂ cake	2 starch
Cake, no icing	¹⁄₁₂ cake, or a 3-in. square	2 starch, 2 fat
Cookies	2 small (1¾ in. across)	1 starch, 1 fat
Frozen fruit yogurt	⅓ cup	1 starch
Gingersnaps	3	1 starch
Granola	¼ cup	1 starch, 1 fat
Granola bars	1 small	1 starch, 1 fat
Ice cream, any flavor	½ cup	1 starch, 2 fat
Ice milk, any flavor	½ cup	1 starch, 1 fat
Sherbet, any flavor	¼ cup	1 starch
Snack chips,* all varieties	1 oz.	1 starch, 2 fat
Vanilla wafers	6 small	1 starch, 1 fat

*If more than one serving is eaten, these foods have 400 milligrams or more of sodium.

PUBLICATIONS OF THE AMERICAN DIABETES ASSOCIATION

Diabetes Forecast, a monthly magazine for people with diabetes and their families. A subscription to *Forecast* is a primary benefit of membership in the ADA for some 225,000 people with diabetes and their families. Over the years, it has helped to improve their quality of life with lively and timely articles on all aspects of living successfully with diabetes.

Diabetes: Reach for Health and Freedom, an informative, accessible guidebook for people with diabetes that emphasizes psychosocial adjustment.

Children with Diabetes, the essential manual for parents and other adults who deal with diabetic children. It covers all the details of diabetes management and takes a sensitive look at the psychological needs of all family members.

The Lifestage Booklets, basic yet comprehensive information about diabetes, targeted to different age groups. The series includes booklets for parents, children, teens/young adults, the middle years, and the later years.

Family Cookbooks, Volumes I and II, economical, kitchen-tested recipes the whole family can enjoy, including exchange values and nutrient breakdowns per serving. Tips on eating out, brown-bagging, weight control, and balancing food and medication for sick days are included. An all-new Volume III, featuring microwave and ethnic cooking, will be available after October 1987.

Holiday Cookbook, traditional holiday favorites adapted to be low in sugar, salt, and fat. More than 175 recipes, with current exchange values and nutrient breakdowns per serving, that the whole family can enjoy during the holidays and year-round.

Exchange Lists for Meal Planning, the definitive guide to creating and maintaining a nutritious and healthy diet, developed by the ADA and the American Dietetic Association. The Exchange Lists reflect the latest scientific findings on good nutrition.

Healthy Food Choices, a simplified version of the *Exchange Lists for Meal Planning,* in poster form.

The ADA also distributes a free, quarterly newsletter with practical advice and helpful hints on living with diabetes. To subscribe, call the number below.

For more information on these publications or how to join the ADA, write or call:

American Diabetes Association
Diabetes Information Service Center
1660 Duke Street
Alexandria, VA 22314
800-ADA-DISC
(In Virginia and Washington, D.C., metro area, dial 703-549-1500.)

THE AMERICAN DIABETES ASSOCIATION AFFILIATES

The American Diabetes Association is the nation's largest voluntary health agency dedicated to finding the cause and cure for diabetes and improving the well-being of all people with diabetes and their families. The ADA carries out this important mission through the efforts of thousands of volunteers working at state affiliates and local chapters in more than 800 communities throughout the United States.

Membership in the ADA puts you in contact with a network of more than 225,000 caring people. Our affiliates and chapters offer support groups, educational programs, counseling, and other special services. Membership in the ADA also brings with it 12 issues of our lively patient education magazine, *Diabetes Forecast*. Each issue is packed with practical information on diabetes management, in an interesting and lively format.

Information on ADA membership and programs is available through the American Diabetes Association, Diabetes Information Service Center, 1660 Duke Street, Alexandria, VA 22314, 800-ADA-DISC. (In Virginia or the Washington, D.C., metro area, dial 703-549-1500.) Or, contact the ADA affiliate in your state, listed below.

Alabama Affiliate, Inc.
904 Bob Wallace Avenue
Suite 222
Huntsville, AL 35801
(205) 533-5775 or (205) 533-5776

Alaska Affiliate, Inc.
201 E. 3rd Avenue
Suite 301
Anchorage, AK 99501
(907) 276-3607

Arizona Affiliate, Inc.
7337 North 19th Avenue
Room 404
Phoenix, AZ 85021
(602) 995-1515

Arkansas Affiliate, Inc.
Tanglewood Shopping Center
7509 Cantrell Road
Suite 227
Little Rock, AR 72207
(501) 666-6345

Northern California Affiliate, Inc.
2550 9th Street
Suite 114
Berkeley, CA 94710
(415) 644-0920

Southern California Affiliate, Inc.
3460 Wilshire Boulevard
Suite 900
Los Angeles, CA 90010
(213) 381-3639

Colorado Affiliate, Inc.
2450 South Downing Street
Denver, CO 80210
(303) 778-7556

Connecticut Affiliate, Inc.
P.O. Box 10160
West Hartford, CT 06110
(203) 249-9942 or (800) 842-6323

Delaware Affiliate, Inc.
2713 Lancaster Avenue
Wilmington, DE 19805
(302) 656-0030

Washington, D.C. Area Affiliate, Inc.
1819 H Street, N.W.
Suite 1200
Washington, DC 20006
(202) 331-8303

Florida Affiliate, Inc.
P.O. Box 19745 (mailing address)
Orlando, FL 32814
3101 Maguire Blvd. (street address)
Suite 288
Orlando, FL 32803
(305) 894-6664

Georgia Affiliate, Inc.
3783 Presidential Parkway
Suite 102
Atlanta, GA 30340
(404) 454-8401

Hawaii Affiliate, Inc.
510 South Beretania Street
Honolulu, HI 96813
(808) 521-5677

Idaho Affiliate, Inc.
1528 Vista
Boise, ID 83705
(208) 342-2774

Downstate Illinois Affiliate, Inc.
965 North Water Street
Decatur, IL 62523
(217) 422-8228

Northern Illinois Affiliate, Inc.
6 North Michigan Avenue
Suite 1202
Chicago, IL 60602
(312) 346-1805

Indiana Affiliate, Inc.
222 South Downey Avenue
Suite 320
Indianapolis, IN 46219
(317) 352-9226

Iowa Affiliate, Inc.
888 Tenth Street
Marion, IA 52302
(319) 373-0530

Kansas Affiliate, Inc.
3210 E. Douglas
Wichita, KS 67208
(316) 681-6091

Kentucky Affiliate, Inc.
P.O. Box 345 (mailing address)
Frankfort, KY 40602
306 West Main (street address)
Suite 513
Frankfort, KY 40602
(502) 223-2971

Louisiana Affiliate, Inc.
9420 Lindale Avenue
Suite B
Baton Rouge, LA 70815
(504) 927-7732

Maine Affiliate, Inc.
59 Northport Avenue
Belfast, ME 04915
(207) 338-5132

Maryland Affiliate, Inc.
3701 Old Court Road
Suite 19
Baltimore, MD 21208
(301) 486-5516

Massachusetts Affiliate, Inc.
190 North Main Street
Natick, MA 01760
(617) 655-6900

Michigan Affiliate, Inc.
The Clausen Bldg. North Unit
23100 Providence Drive
Suite 475
Southfield, MI 48075
(313) 552-0480

Minnesota Affiliate, Inc.
3005 Ottawa Avenue, South
Minneapolis, MN 55416
(612) 920-6796

Mississippi Affiliate, Inc.
10 Lakeland Circle
Jackson, MS 39216
(601) 981-9511

Missouri Affiliate, Inc.
P.O. Box 11
Columbia, MO 65201
(314) 443-8611

Montana Affiliate, Inc.
Box 2411 (mailing address)
Great Falls, MT 59403
600 Central Plaza (street address)
Suite 304
Great Falls, MT 59401
(406) 761-0908

Nebraska Affiliate, Inc.
2730 S. 114th St.
Omaha, NE 68144
(402) 391-1251

Nevada Affiliate, Inc.
4550 East Charleston Boulevard
Las Vegas, NV 89104
(702) 459-7099

New Hampshire Affiliate, Inc.
P.O. Box 595 (mailing address)
Manchester, NH 03105
104 Middle Street (street address)
Manchester, NH 03101
(603) 627-9579

New Jersey Affiliate, Inc.
P.O. Box 6423 (mailing address)
312 North Adamsville Rd. (street
address)
Bridgewater, NJ 08807
(201) 725-7878

New Mexico Affiliate, Inc.
525 San Pedro, N.E.
Suite 101
Albuquerque, NM 87108
(505) 266-5716

New York Diabetes Affiliate, Inc.
505 8th Avenue
New York, NY 10018
(212) 947-9707

New York State Affiliate, Inc.
P.O. Box 1037 (mailing address)
Syracuse, NY 13201
113 East Willow Street (street
address)
Syracuse, NY 13202
(315) 472-9111

North Carolina Affiliate, Inc.
2315-A Sunset Avenue
Rocky Mount, NC 27801
(919) 937-4121

North Dakota Affiliate, Inc.
P.O. Box 234 (mailing address)
Grand Forks, ND 58206-0234
101 North 3rd Street (street address)
Suite 502
Grand Forks, ND 58201
(701) 746-4427

Ohio Affiliate, Inc.
1855 Fountain Square Court
Suite 310
Columbus, OH 43224-1360
(614) 263-2330

Oklahoma Affiliate, Inc.
Warren Professional Building
6465 South Yale Avenue
Suite 423
Tulsa, OK 74136
(918) 492-3839 or (800) 722-5448

Oregon Affiliate, Inc.
3607 S.W. Corbett Street
Portland, OR 97201
(503) 228-0849

Greater Philadelphia Affiliate, Inc.
21 South Fifth Street
The Bourse
Suite 570
Philadelphia, PA 19106
(215) 627-7718

Western Pennsylvania Affiliate, Inc.
4617 Winthrop Street
Pittsburgh, PA 15213
(412) 682-3392

Mid-Pennsylvania Affiliate, Inc.
2045 Westgate Drive
Suite B-1
Bethlehem, PA 18017
(215) 867-6660

Rhode Island Affiliate, Inc.
4 Fallon Avenue
Providence, RI 02908
(401) 331-0099

South Carolina Affiliate, Inc.
P.O. Box 50782
Columbia, SC 29250
(803) 799-4246

South Dakota Affiliate, Inc.
P.O. Box 659
Sioux Falls, SD 57101
(605) 335-7670

Tennessee Affiliate, Inc.
1701 21st Avenue, South
Room 403
Nashville, TN 37212
(615) 298-9919

Texas Affiliate, Inc.
8140 North Mopac
Building 1
Suite 130
Austin, TX 78759
(512) 343-6981

Utah Affiliate, Inc.
564 East 300 South
Salt Lake, UT 84102
(801) 363-3024

Vermont Affiliate, Inc.
217 Church Street
Burlington, VT 05401
(802) 862-3882

Virginia Affiliate, Inc.
404 8th Street, N.E.
Suite C
Charlottesville, VA 22901
(804) 293-4953

Washington Affiliate, Inc.
3201 Fremont Avenue North
Seattle, WA 98103
(206) 632-4576

West Virginia Affiliate, Inc.
Professional Building
1036 Quarrier Street
Room 404
Charleston, WV 25301
(304) 346-6418 or (800) 642-3055

Wisconsin Affiliate, Inc.
10721 West Capitol Drive
Milwaukee, WI 53222
(414) 464-9395

Wyoming Affiliate, Inc.
2908 Kelly Drive
Cheyenne, WY 82001
(307) 638-3578

BIBLIOGRAPHY

General References

Hamburg, B. A., L. F. Lipsett, G. E. Inoff, and A. L. Drash, eds. 1979. *Behavioral and Psychosocial Issues in Diabetes, Proceedings of the National Conference.* Washington, D.C.: U.S. Dept. Health & Human Services.

Leptich, J. 1980. "Positive outlook aids Montreal's Gullickson in coping with diabetes." *Chicago Suburban Tribune,* June 23.

Podolsky, S., ed. 1980. *Clinical Diabetes: Modern Management.* New York: Appleton-Century-Croft.

Rifkin, H., and P. Raskin, eds. 1981. *Diabetes Mellitus. Vol. 5.* Bowie: American Diabetes Associates, Robert J. Brady Company.

Talbert, W. 1975. "Testimony presented to the National Diabetes Commission on diabetes." *Report of the National Commission on Diabetes to the Congress of the U.S.,* Vol. 2, Part 1, Public Testimony, May 1.

West, J. 1978. *Epidemiology of Diabetes and Its Vascular Lesions.* New York: Elsevier.

Research References

Anderson, J. W., and B. Sieling. 1981. "High-fiber diets for diabetics: Unconventional but effective." *Geriatrics* 36 (5).

Blackshear, P. J., T. D. Rhode, F. Prosl, and H. Buchwald. 1979. "The implantable infusion pump: A new concept in drug delivery." In *Medical Progress through Technology.* New York: Springer-Verlag.

Cooper, A. R., ed. 1980. "Development of novel semipermeable tubular membranes for a hybrid artificial pancreas." In *Ultrafiltration Membranes and Applications.* New York: Plenum Publishing Corp.

Craighead, J. E. 1981. "Viral diabetes mellitus in man and experimental animals." *American Journal of Medicine* 70 (1): 127–34.

Lacy, P. E., J. M. Davie, and E. H. Finke. 1981. "Transplantation of insulin-producing tissue." *American Journal of Medicine* 70 (3).

Lee, S. M., and R. Bressler. 1981. "Prevention of diabetic nephropathy by diet control in the db/db mouse." *Diabetes: The Journal of the American Diabetes Association* 30 (2).

Schade, D. S., R. P. Eaton, and W. Spencer. 1981. "Implantation of an artificial pancreas." *Journal of the American Medical Association* 245 (7).

GLOSSARY OF MEDICAL TERMS

Acetone: fragments of fatty acid formed during the abnormal metabolism of body fat

Adrenal: a gland of the endocrine system that produces many essential hormones, including adrenalin and cortisone

Albumin: a water-soluble protein present in the urine under certain conditions

Alpha cells: cells in the pancreas that produce the hormone glucagon

Amniocentesis: a test of the amniotic fluid surrounding the fetus, made to help determine the health of the baby

Aneurysm: a bulging or ballooning out of a blood vessel wall

Angiogram: a series of rapid X rays of a blood vessel made after a dye has been injected into the blood vessels

Angiopathy: disease of the blood vessels

Antibiotic: a drug with the capacity to help destroy bacteria in the body

Antibodies: substances occurring naturally in the blood that help fight infection in the body

Arteriosclerosis: a thickening, hardening, and loss of elasticity of the blood vessels, particularly the arteries

Artery: a blood vessel that carries blood away from the heart

Atherosclerosis: a form of arteriosclerosis in which deposits of calcium and fatlike substances are formed in and on the lining of the blood vessels

Athlete's foot: a fungus infection of the feet

ATPase: an enzyme found in body cells that is essential for normal energy production

Autonomic: involuntary, self-controlling

Basement membrane: a thin layer underlying the inner lining of the blood vessel walls

Beta cells: the insulin-producing cells of the pancreas

Biosynthetic: referring to production of a chemical compound by a living organism

Bladder: sac where urine is stored until released by the body

Blood pressure: the force exerted by blood as it is pumped through the arteries

Blood sugar: the sugar formed in the digestive process, which circulates in the blood as glucose

Blood vessel: arteries, veins, and smaller vessles that make up the circulatory network to carry blood throughout the body

Bronchitis: inflammation of the bronchial tubes

Candidiasis: a yeastlike fungus infection

Capillaries: tiny blood vessels that connect the smallest arteries to the smallest veins in the body tissues

Cardiovascular: pertaining to the heart and blood vessels

Cataract: an opaque film in the lens of the eye

Cell: the microscopic unit of structure that forms the basis of all living things

Cementum: a thin layer of bone that helps to support the roots of the teeth

Cholesterol: a fatlike substance normally produced in the human body and also found in animal tissue

Chronic: of long duration, continuing

Coma: loss of consciousness

Conjunctiva: the outer lining of the eyeball

Cornea: the clear, transparent center of the eye through which light enters

Cortisone: a hormone produced by the adrenal gland

Coxsackie: a group of viruses, usually causing a variety of mild infections, and named for the place where they were first identified

Cranial: pertaining to the skull

Cystitis: an inflammation of the urinary bladder

Dehydration: loss of water or fluid from the body or tissues

Dermopathy: any disease of the skin

Diabetologist: a doctor skilled in the treatment of diabetes

Diarrhea: frequent, loose, watery stools

Emphysema: a chronic lung disease characterized by enlargement of the air sacs of the lungs

Enzyme: a protein produced by living cells that enhances the chemical reactions involved in body metabolism

Estriol: a hormone produced by the fetus and placenta during pregnancy

Exocrine gland: a gland that produces substances necessary for body funtion, such as the digestive enzymes and those secretions carried by ducts and tubules

Fetus: the developing, unborn baby

Fluorophotometer: an electronic instrument that measures circulation of blood in the eye when a dye has been injected into the blood vessels

Fungus: a vegetative plant that subsists/lives on dead or living tissue

Gangrene: death of body tissue, usually caused by a lack of blood supply

Gene: unit of inheritance found in all living cells

Generic drug: a term used to indicate drugs of a certain class or family

Gestational: referring to the period of pregnancy from conception to birth

Gingivae: the gums that surround the teeth

Gingivitis: inflammation of the gums

Gland: a body cell, or group of body cells, that produce secretions frequently used elsewhere in the body

Glomeruli: tiny tufts of blood vessels that help to make up the functional unit of structure of the kidneys

Glomerulosclerosis: hardening of the glomeruli

Glucagon: a hormone produced in the pancreas that raises the level of blood sugar

Glucose: a form of sugar; blood sugar

Glycogen: a form of glucose stored in the liver and muscles

Glycosuria: the presence of glucose in the urine

Glycosylated hemoglobin: glucose chemically bound to the hemoglobin of red blood cells

Gonads: glands of the male and female endocrine systems that produce the sex hormones

Hemodialysis: treatment used to cleanse the blood by passing it through an artificial kidney mechanism

Hemoglobin: the iron-protein chemical matter of red blood cells which functions in carrying oxygen from the lungs to the body tissues

Hemorrhage: uncontrolled bleeding from a broken blood vessel

Hormone: a chemical substance produced by body cells which produces a specific stimulating effect on other body cells

Hyperglycemia: a blood sugar level of higher than normal limits

Hyperinsulinemia: an excessive amount of insulin in the blood

Hyperosmolar: characterized by high blood sugar, excess fluid in the body, and extreme dehydration

Hypertension: high blood pressure

Hypoglycemia: a blood sugar level of lower than normal limits

Immune system: naturally produced substances in the body that help to overcome disease and infection

Implant: any material or device inserted or grafted into the body, usually to improve bodily function

Impotence: the inability in males, to start, sustain, or complete the act of sexual intercourse

Insulin: a hormone produced by the pancreas that lowers blood sugar

Ischemia: a local and temporary lack of adequate blood supply to a body part

Islets of Langerhans: clusters of cells in the pancreas which include the insulin-producing beta cells

Ketoacidosis (ketosis): the presence of ketones in the blood which have spilled over into the urine, an indication that diabetes is out of control

Ketones: chemical fragments of fatty acids caused by the incomplete burning of body fat for energy, found in the urine under certain conditions

Kidneys: organs that filter blood and chemical wastes in the body

Lipohypertrophies: raised toughened areas of the skin

Lipotrophies: deep indentations in the skin

Liver: a large glandular organ located in the upper abdomen, whose function is vital to many body processes

Macroangiopathy: a disease of the large blood vessels

Metabolism: the sum total of all physical and chemical changes taking place in the body, including the processing of food for repair and maintenance of body tissue, and for use as energy

Microangiopathy: a disease of the small blood vessels

Moniliasis: a yeastlike fungus infection of the skin

Necrobiosis lipoidica diabeticorum: a skin disease sometimes occurring in diabetes, characterized by dark red spots on the shins that can crack open and become painful

Nephropathy: disease of the kidneys

Nephrosclerosis: a hardening of the blood vessels of the kidneys

Neuropathy: any disease of the nerves

Obesity: the condition of overweight

Oral hypoglycemic compounds: drugs taken by mouth that stimulate the release of insulin in the body

Pancreas: a glandular organ located behind the stomach, having both endocrine and exocrine tissue and function

Paralysis: a loss of voluntary muscle control

Pelvis of the kidney: a cavity within each kidney that helps collect and channel urine to the ureters

Periodontal: referring to the tissue and bone surrounding the teeth

Photocoagulation: a scarring made with an intense light to seal off a broken blood vessel

Pituitary: an endocrine gland at the base of the brain that produces many hormones which directly affect many body functions

Placenta: a membrane attached to the lining of the uterus that encloses and provides nourishment to the fetus

Plaque: a film formed on the teeth by food, saliva, and bacteria

Plasma: the liquid portion of the blood

Podiatrist: a doctor who specializes in the treatment of foot disorders

Pyelitis: inflammation of the pelvic area

Pyelonephritis: inflammation of the kidney pelvis and glomeruli

Pyorrhea: a disease of the gums characterized by a shrinking away of the gums from the teeth

Receptor: a sensitive area on a body cell

Renal: pertaining to the kidneys

Retina: the light- and image-sensitive area on the inside of the eye

Retinopathy: disease of the retina of the eye

Serum: the clear liquid part of the blood which appears after clotting

Sign: something that can be seen; obvious evidence of a disease or condition

Somogyi effect: a rebound effect in diabetics of low and high blood sugar caused by too much insulin; named after the doctor who first identified it

Stroke: a paralysis caused by damage to the brain cells

Stye: an infection of the eyelid

Superior vena cava: the main vein leading to the heart

Symptom: something that is felt; any conscious change in body function

Syndrome: a combination or group of signs or symptoms

Thyroid: an endocrine gland located in the base of the neck that produces hormones vital to normal growth, development, and metabolism of the body cells

Transplant: the transfer of a living organ or tissue from one part to another, or from one individual to another

Trimester: a three-month period of pregnancy

Ulcer: an open sore of the skin

Ultrasonic probe: a noninvasive test performed with an instrument that detects sounds and movements inside the body

Ureters: tubes that carry urine from the kidneys to the bladder

Urinary tract: organs and ducts of the body (kidneys, ureters, urethra, and bladder) that secrete and eliminate urine

Urine: secretion of the kidneys

Vascular: pertaining to the blood vessels

Vein: a blood vessel that carries blood to the heart

Viruses: living organisms that can cause many diseases, including measles, mumps, and hepatitis

Vitrectomy: a surgical procedure performed to restore eyesight lost due to vitreous hemorrhage and retinal detachment

Vitreous: the fluid-filled chamber in the center of the eye

Void: to urinate

INDEX

A

ADA, *see* American Diabetes Association
Adjustment, to diabetes, 18–21
Adolescents, diabetes in, 140–141, 147–148
Adult-onset diabetes, *see* Non-insulin-dependent diabetes
Aerobic exercises, 40
Alcohol, 57–59
  effect of, on body, 57–58
American Diabetes Association (ADA), 4, 5, 26, 29, 62, 64, 84, 156, 173–178
  address, 174, 175
  formation, 3–4
Arteriosclerosis, 123
Aspartame, 29
Atherosclerosis, 24
ATPase, in obesity, 114–115
Autonomic neuropathy, 135–136

B

Background retinopathy, 128
Basic meal plan, 157–159
Beta cells
  immunosuppression and, 152
  in obesity, 114
  in transplants, 153
Blood glucose
  fiber and, 154

normal readings of, 13, 32, 97
response to meal, 15–17
self-monitoring of, 29, 30, 151
Blood glucose tolerance test, 13
Blood tests, 29–33
  keeping records of, 94–95
  mechanics of, 31
  products used in, 31
  urine tests versus, 29–30
Blood vessel disease, 122–126
  gangrene, 126
  ischemia, 124
  legs and feet and, 124
  prevention, 126
  treatment for, 124–126
Body weight, computing desirable level of, 115
Borderline diabetes, 9–10

C

Calories, 24–25
  caloric equivalents of physical exercise, 44–45
  in daily meal plan, 26
Carbohydrate diet, for diabetes, 2
Carbohydrates, 23
  in meal plan, 26
Career choices, diabetics and, 142
Careers and employment, 61–65
  changing, 63–64
  discrimination in, 64–65
Cell receptors, in obesity, 114
Cholesterol, 24, 155

Controlling diabetes, 13–17
   guidelines for, 16–17
Council on Exercise, 6
Cranial neuropathy, 137
Crisis times, in lives of diabetics,
   139–140
Cystitis, 133

D

Dental problems, 48–51
Diabetes, cause of, 10–12
Diabetes in life stages, 144–150
   adolescence, 147–148
   early childhood, 144–145
   elderly, 149–150
   elementary years, 147–148
   middle age, 149
   young adulthood, 148
Diabetic coma, 108–111
Diabetic dermopathy, 52
Diabetic diarrhea, 136
Diabetic nephropathy, 131–133
Diabetic neuropathy, *see* Neuropathy
Diabetic retinopathy, 128–131
   prevention, 131
Diet prescription, 116–119
Diets, for diabetes, 2
   goals of, 5
   importance of, 22–26
Double vision, 128
Driving, diabetics and, 60–61

E

Elderly, diabetes in, 142–143,
   149–150
Employment, *see* Careers and employment
Energy production, 7–8
Enzymes, 114
Estriol, 76
Exchange Lists for Meal Planning,
   4–5, 26–29, 154, 155, 159–173

combination foods, 171–172
fat list, 168–169
free foods, 170–171
fruit list, 165–167
meat list, 161–164
milk list, 167–168
starch/bread list, 159–161
vegetable list, 164–165
Exercise, 5–6, 39–45
   caloric equivalents of physical exercise, 44–45
   when traveling, 71
   weight control and, 119
Eye, 127
   minor problems of, 127–128

F

Family, 138–143
   counseling, 140–142
   psychosocial issues, 138–139
   resolving conflicts, 139–140
Fat, 23–24
   in meal plan, 26
Feet, care of, 45–48
Fiber, 23, 154–155
Food diary, 116–117
Foods for occasional use, 172–173
Fructose, 29
Fungus infections, 52

G

Genetics, research on, 152
Gestational diabetes, 9
Gingivitis, 49
Glomerulosclerosis, 132
Glucagon, 7, 99–104
   administering, 103–104
   forms of, 104
   general directions for use,
     99–100
   preparations for injection,
     100–102
Glucose, 7

Glucose tolerance test curves, 14
Glycemic index, 155
Glycogen, 7
Glycosylated hemoglobin A₁C, 36

H

Hemodialysis, 133
Hemoglobin A₁C, 36
Hemorrhage, of eye, 128
Heredity, and development of diabetes, 10
High renal threshold, 30
Historical perspective, on diabetes, 1–6
Hyperglycemia, 16
  signs of, 111
Hyperinsulinism, 114
Hyperosmolar coma, 55; *see also* Hyperosmolar nonketotic coma
Hyperosmolar nonketotic coma, 111–112
Hypoglycemia, 4, 16
  hyperglycemia compared with, 110
  symptoms, 110
Hypoglycemic reaction, *see* Insulin reaction

I

Illness, 53–56
  diet during, 54–55
  testing blood and urine during, 53–54
  tips for, 56
Immunology, research on, 152
Immunosuppression, 152
Impaired glucose tolerance, 9–10
Implantable glucose sensor/pump, 153–154
Impotence, 136–137
Incidence, of diabetes, 1
Indian tribes, diabetes in, 12
Inheritance, of diabetes, 73

Insulin, 7
  action of, 82–83
  action time, 79
  cost, 81–82
  discovery of, 3
  duration of, 79
  injection techniques, 84–91
  lipohypertrophies from, 89
  lipotrophies from, 89
  measurement of, in blood, 4
  mixing of, for injections, 91–94
  onset, 79
  peak, 79
  purity of, 81
  source of, 81
  storage of, 94
  syringe for, 83, 94
  in Type II diabetes, 121
  types of, 80–81
Insulin-dependence, exercise and, 41–42
Insulin-dependent diabetes, 8–9
Insulin-dependent Type I person, 111
Insulin pump, 75, 83–84, 151
Insulin reaction, 94–107
  carbohydrates in, 104
  cause of 96–97, 106
  diabetic coma versus, 108–109
  glucagon for, 99–104
  prevention of, 104–105
  symptoms, 97, 106–107
  as term, 108–109
  treatment for, 98–99, 107
  unconsciousness and, 104, 107
Insulin resistance, 4
  research in, 155
Insurance, for diabetics, 65–67
  group plans, 65–66
  term insurance, 66
  whole life insurance, 66
Islets of Langerhans, 2

J

Juvenile-onset diabetes, *see* Insulin-dependent diabetes

K

Ketoacidosis, 53–55, 108–111
  symptoms, 111
  treatment, 108
Ketones, 53–55, 107
  testing for, 35
Kidney disease, 131–133
  prevention, 134
  treatment, 133–134
Kidney transplants, 134

L

L insulin, 80
Laser therapy, 151
Latent diabetes, 10
Lente, 3, 80
Life stages, *see* Diabetes in life
  stages

M

Macroangiopathy, 122, 123
Madison Conference, 139–140
Marijuana, 59–60
Marriage, of diabetics, 142
Marriage and pregnancy, 73–76
  inheritance of diabetes and,
    73–74
  pregnancy, 74–76
Maturity-onset diabetes, *see*
    Non-insulin-dependent diabe-
    tes
Meal plan, 26, 78–79
Microangiopathy, 122
  prevention, 123
Minerals, 24
  supplements of, 25
Molecular binding, 155
Monounsaturated fats, 24
Motor neuropathy, 137

N

N insulin, 80

National Diabetes Research and
  Education Act of 1974, 4
National Institute of Health, 156
Necrobiosis lipoidica diabeticorum,
  52–53
Nephrosclerosis, 133
Neuropathic ulcers, 135
Neuropathy, 134–137
  impotence in, 136–137
Non-insulin-dependent diabetes, 9
  causes of, 11
NPH insulin, 3, 80
Nutrition, 154–155

O

Obesity, 11, 12, 113–116
  ATPase in, 114–115
  causes of, 114
  cell receptors of, 114
  control of, 115–116
  definition, 114
  research on, 155
Oral hypoglycemic compounds,
  119–121
  action times of, 120
  interaction with other drugs,
    120–121

P

Pancreas, 2, 7
  transplant, 153
Periodontal disease, 48–51
Peripheral neuropathy, 52, 135
Photocoagulation, 129–130
Physical inactivity, as cause of dia-
  betes, 11–12
PIMS, *see* Programmable implant-
  able medication system
Polynesian population, diabetes in,
  12
Polyunsaturated fats, 24
  in meal plan, 26
Pregnancy, 74–76
  as cause of diabetes, 11

Programmable implantable medication system (PIMS), 154
Proliferative retinopathy, 128–129
Protein, 23
  in meal plan, 25
Pyelitis, 133
Pyelonephritis, 133
Pyorrhea, 49
PZI insulin, 81

R

Renal threshold, 32–33
Research, 151–156
  on genetics, 152
  on immunology, 152
  on implantable glucose
    sensor/pumps, 153–154
  on insulin resistance, 155
  on nutrition, 154–155
  on obesity, 155

S

Saccharin, 29
Saturated fats, 24
  in meal plan, 26
Secondary diabetes, 10
Self-monitoring, of blood glucose, 151
Semilente, 80
Skin problems, 51–53
Smoking, 59–60
Somogyi effect, 107–108
Sorbitol, 29
Stress, 10–12, 36–39
  definition, 36
  effect of, on body, 37–38
  reduction of, 38–39
Stress test, 42
Sugar, 28–29
  names of, 28
Symptoms, of diabetes, 12–13
Symposium on Diabetes and Exercise, 5–6

T

Transplants, 152–153
Travel, 67–72
  diabetes schedule and, 71–72
  eating and drinking away from
    home, 72
  exercise, 71
  packing for, 69–70
  preparation for, 67–69
  tips for insulin users, 70–71
Type I, insulin-dependent diabetes,
    77–95; *see also*
    Insulin-dependent diabetes
  diet and, 25
  exercise and, 40–41
  inheritance of, 73
  insulin in, 79–95
  meal plan for, 78–79
  self-management of, 94–95
  self-monitoring of, 30
  treatment goals, 77–79
  urine tests and, 35
Type II, non-insulin-dependent diabetes, 113–121; *see also*
    Non-insulin-dependent diabetes
  diet and, 25
  exercise and, 42
  hyperosmolar coma in, 55
  inheritance of, 73
  insulin in, 121
  self-monitoring of, 30
  treatment goals, 113–114
  urine tests and, 34, 35

U

U insulin, 81
Ultralente, 81
Urinary tract infections, 133
Urine, ketones in, 53–55, 107
Urine tests, 33–36
  blood tests versus, 29–30
  collection in, 34
  keeping records of, 94–95
  timing in, 35
  variety of, 34–35

V

Viral infections, 10
Visual problems, 127–131
Vitamins, 24
  supplements of, 25
Vitrectomy, 130

W

Weight control, exercise and, 119
Weight loss
  food diary for, 116–117
  tips for, 116–118
Women, with diabetes, 151